Roth

The Radiology of Acute Cervical Spine Trauma

Second Edition

The Radiology of Acute Cervical Spine Trauma

Second Edition

John H. Harris, Jr., M.D., D.Sc.

Professor and Chairman
Department of Radiology
University of Texas Medical School
Houston, Texas

Beth Edeiken-Monroe, M.D.

Assistant Professor
Chief of Diagnosis
Department of Radiology
University of Texas Medical School
Houston, Texas

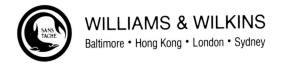

WILLIAMS & WILKINS
Baltimore • Hong Kong • London • Sydney

Editor: Timothy R. Grayson
Associate Editor: Carol Eckhart
Copy Editor: Deborah K. Tourtlotte
Design: JoAnne Janowiak
Illustration Planning: Lorraine Wrzosek
Production: Anne G. Seitz

Copyright © 1987
Williams & Wilkins
428 East Preston Street
Baltimore, MD 21202, U.S.A.

Accurate indications, adverse reactions, and dosage schedules for drugs are provided in this book, but it is possible that they may change. The reader is urged to review the package information data of the manufacturers of the medications mentioned.

Printed in the United States of America
First Edition, 1978

Library of Congress Cataloging-in-Publication Data

Harris, John H. Jr., 1925–
  The radiology of acute cervical spine trauma.

  Bibliography: p.
  Includes index.
  1. Vertebrae, Cervical–Wounds and injuries.
2. Vertebrae, Cervical–Radiography.   I. Edeiken-Monroe,
Beth.   II. Title. [DNLM: 1. Cervical Vertebrae–
injuries.   2. Cervical Vertebrae–radiography.
WE 725 H314r]
RD533.H37   1987   617′.375044   86-22424
ISBN 0-683-03928-8

90 91 92   10 9 8 7 6 5 4

To our fathers
John H. Harris, M.D. (deceased)
Jack Edeiken, M.D.
who guided, taught, and inspire us
and to
Cathy and Matt
who tolerate, encourage, and
support us with their love.

Foreword

Skeletal trauma is one of the most serious disorders affecting mankind. Such trauma occurs at all ages, in every country in the world, and particularly in those areas where physical violence inflicted on humans is a commonplace occurrence. Injuries to the skeleton are encountered most frequently in highly industrialized countries, principally where the motor vehicle is an important mode of transportation, such as in the United States. Although trauma to any part of the skeleton may occur, injuries to the spine, and particularly the cervical spine, constitute one of the leading causes of disability.

The second edition of this extremely informative work by John Harris and Beth Edeiken Monroe (the first edition was published in 1978, with Dr. Harris as the sole author) has within its content all of the relevant information necessary for radiologists and orthopaedic and neurological clinicians to deal with virtually any patient who has sustained an acute injury to the cervical spine.

The work is divided into 11 chapters; an outline of the basic content of each chapter follows:

Chapter 1 is a long introduction to normal anatomy and embryology; it is beautifully illustrated and replete with anatomical sketches and illustrative radiological material. The various techniques used in the examination of the cervical spine are described, with particular emphasis on plain films and computerized tomography. The normal anatomy of the soft tissues of the cervical spine also is considered.

Chapter 2 is a continuation of the technical studies used, principally relating to the various imaging techniques. Particular attention is paid to the acutely traumatized patient, but the techniques applicable to the less severely injured patient are also described. The various modalities used are discussed in depth. These include plain-film tomography, three-dimensional computed tomography (3-D CT), myelography, ultrasonography, and imaging with magnetic resonance (MR).

Three-dimensional computerized tomography is considered, with a description of specially designed software necessary for this type of study. Three-D CT allows rotation of images about any axis and permits transection of images along axial, coronal, and saggital planes. The authors illustrate that 3-D CT represents a more comprehensive method of imaging complex injuries and demonstrate that, in some instances, 3-D CT is far superior to standard CT. This method is shown to be specifically indicated in injuries to the posterior arch and in cases where plain films and multiplanar CT studies are inconsistent with the clinical findings.

A short section on the efficacy of myelography in trauma to the cervical

FOREWORD

spine is included. Although myelography is now considerably limited, the authors demonstrate the applicability of the myelogram in certain traumatic situations.

The use of ultrasonography in acute injuries to the cervical spine is discussed. Indeed, the applicability of ultrasonography in such instances is extremely limited, but the authors describe the use of intraoperative real-time monitoring with ultrasound for the reduction of "burst" fractures. Such monitoring requires laminectomy, giving important information about the position of spinal fragments and perhaps, even delineating hematomas of the spinal cord.

In the same chapter, a short section stresses imaging with magnetic resonance, which at the present time is limited in acute trauma to the cervical spine, but promises to be of great help in assessing trauma to the spinal cord.

Chapter 3 includes a practical and highly useful classification of acute trauma to the cervical spine; the mechanisms of the various injuries are described in detail. An understanding of the seven major types of injuries to the cervical spine described in this chapter provides vital information. Each of the following seven chapters deals with a major type of injury as outlined in Chapter 3, and the various mechanisms of injuries are discussed in detail:

Chapter 4—*flexion* injuries in which five varieties are named and discussed; Chapter 5—unilateral facetal dislocations; Chapter 6—simultaneous hyperextension and rotation injuries (pillar fracture); Chapter 7—vertical compression injuries, which are further subdivided into Jefferson fractures of the atlas and bursting fractures of the lower cervical spine; Chapter 8—hyperextension injuries, which are subdivided into seven types; Chapter 9—lateral flexion injuries, producing fractures of the uncinate process; and Chapter 10–injuries of diverse or poorly understood mechanisms, which include occipitoatlantal disassociation, three types of fractures of the odontoid process, acute traumatic rotatory atlantoaxial dislocation, torticollis (associated with atlantoaxial rotatory displacement), and subtle cervicocranial injuries.

The final chapter (11) is an excellent description of anomalies and normal variants of the cervical spine that may simulate fracture. This chapter is a particularly valuable addition to this work.

In all instances, the working classification provided is truly pragmatic, the mechanisms of injuries are described in depth with great clarity, and the illustrative material is superb. Excellent sketches are appended where necessary.

This book constitutes a major revision of the first edition of the work, with a considerable amount of new discussion, illustrations, and sketches. Of particular interest is the description of 3-D CT in studying trauma of the cervical spine. The authors have written a highly important and significant work, which in this modern era of violence, particularly associated with motor vehicular accidents, should be studied by all physicians who deal with trauma to the cervical spine. A complex subject has been simplified greatly in this well-organized and lucid presentation.

This work is a *must* for radiologists, orthopaedic clinicians, neurologists, neurosurgeons and medical students.

It is a privilege to have been asked to write this foreword.

Harold G. Jacobson, M.D.

Preface to the Second Edition

The reception afforded the first edition of *The Radiology of Acute Cervical Spine Trauma* has been an extreme personal compliment and an extraordinary reward for the effort that went into its preparation and publication.

Since its publication in 1978, readers have kindly made suggestions for improving the text. Most of these have been incorporated in this edition.

In 1980, I was fortunate enough to join the faculty of The University of Texas Medical School at Houston and the staff of the Hermann Hospital, a major trauma center. These affiliations have provided a unique opportunity to be associated with a remarkable group of dedicated, concerned, academically talented and curious traumatologists, orthopaedists, and neurosurgeons in the initial evaluation and management of literally thousands of patients with *acute* cervical spine trauma. An indication of the magnitude of this experience may be gained from the fact that approximately 11,000 patients with acute cervical spine injury have been examined radiographically in the Emergency Center of the Hermann Hospital since July, 1980. Approximately 606 patients with acute cervical spine and/or cord injury have been discharged from Hermann Hospital during the same period.

The concepts of acute cervical spine injury described in the first edition of this text have been enhanced, expanded, clarified, and refined as a result of this experience and as the result of the challenges to definition, description, and illustration demanded by eagerly inquisitive radiology house officers and those of other disciplines as well.

The common use of computed tomography and the developing application of three-dimensional CT reformation and magnetic resonance imaging in the evaluation of acute cervical spine injury have provided new insights and greater understanding into the pathology of trauma of the cervical spine and the cervical cord. These have been included in this revision.

Preface to the Second Edition

The extensive revisions contained in the second edition represent our current understanding of acute cervical spine injury based on the experience and motivation provided by this unique venue. However, we realize that the practice of medicine is an educational continuum driven, in part, by technologic and scientific advances. Therefore, we fully expect subsequent revisions to reflect increased knowledge and understanding based on these advances.

As with the first edition of this text, it remains our intention and sincere hope that this edition will be a useful and ready resource for all those concerned with the evaluation and management of patients with acute cervical spine injury. We hope that it will be a source of explanation and understanding for those wishing to increase their knowledge of these injuries.

Most importantly it is our earnest hope that the patient who has sustained an acute cervical spine injury is the ultimate beneficiary of our efforts.

JHH JR
BSE-M

Preface to the First Edition

The management of acute cervical spine injury begins with the correct roentgen diagnosis of the lesion.

The roentgen diagnosis of acute injuries of the cervical spine depends upon the appropriate radiographic projections obtained in a sequence commensurate with the severity of injury and the clinical condition of the patient. Beyond this, the roentgen diagnosis requires a knowledge of the radiographic anatomy of the cervical spine, particularly its posterior elements, an understanding of the physiology of the normal movements of the cervical spine, and an awareness of the mechanism of injury of the various types of traumatic lesions that may involve the cervical region.

The purpose of this book is to describe and illustrate the radiographic aspects of acute cervical spine trauma. It is readily apparent that there is not a uniformity of opinion in the existing medical literature regarding the etiology and roentgen appearance of all acute injuries of the cervical spine, and it is freely acknowledged that there may be disagreement with some of the content material of this text. However, the concepts presented here do reflect the consensus of an extensive review of the literature relating to acute cervical spine trauma as well as the experience gained through a broad personal involvement in the roentgen evaluation of patients with acute cervical spine injuries.

This work was born of the frustration engendered by the lack of a ready source of reference for assistance in the evaluation of acute cervical spine injuries as encountered in a busy general practice of radiology. It is designed to ameliorate similar frustrations which might be experienced by other radiologists, orthopaedists and neurosurgeons, emergency physicians, and others involved in the diagnosis and management of patients with acute cervical spine injury.

It is sincerely hoped that this effort leads, not only to improved physician knowledge and understanding but, more importantly, to improved patient care.

JHH Jr

Acknowledgments

This page affords the author an opportunity to extend public thanks to those whose interest and efforts have contributed in a major way to the successful completion of the work.

In that context, I am particularly proud to introduce Beth S. Edeiken-Monroe, M.D., as my associate and co-author. Dr. Edeiken-Monroe is third in a line of distinguished radiologists. Her grandfather, Louis Edeiken, M.D., earned a respected reputation in the private practice of radiology during the preeminence of radiology in Philadelphia during the 1930s–1950s. Her father, Jack Edeiken, M.D., currently Professor of Radiology at M.D. Anderson Hospital and Tumor Institute and an international authority in skeletal radiology, needs no introduction to readers of this text.

While Dr. Edeiken-Monroe is known primarily as a teacher of radiology and while she continues to be an excellent, versatile general radiologist, she has become expert in the area of emergency radiology and has developed a particular interest in acute cervical spine injury. This revision could not have been completed without her active assistance and participation.

Millicent Williams has provided valuable library and editorial support. Rosalind Vecchio, Lew Hondros, and Jay David Johnson, B.S., Radiology Department photographers have provided the great majority of the illustrations. A major strength of this text is the high quality of the illustrations that demonstrate the soft tissues and the skeleton equally well. That the illustrations achieve this goal so uniformly is testimony to Mr. Johnson's ability.

High quality illustrations begin with high quality radiographs. In emergency radiology, the radiographic examination is frequently performed under the most difficult clinical circumstances. In the Hermann Hospital, the emergency radiology section is staffed by a group of loyal, dedicated, and exceptionally talented technologists under the supervision of Susan Kaylor, R.T. and includes Elizabeth Berry, Hal

Dunkirk, Ron Whitehead, Ahmad Sadiki, Shailesh Patel, Angela Brisaffe, Jackie North, and Marsha Smith.

The officers and staff of Williams & Wilkins have, as is characteristic of that distinguished publishing house, provided strong support, valuable advice, and patient encouragement during the preparation of the manuscript. Specifically, Sara Finnegan, President, George Stamathis, Senior Editor, Carol Eckhart, Associate Editor, and Anne Seitz, Production Sponsor have earned and deserve my deepest appreciation. During the final months of text preparation, Ms. Finnegan, Ms. Eckhart, and Ms. Seitz have extended themselves and the facilities of Williams & Wilkins, and Waverly Press, Inc. well beyond that traditionally expected of each of these institutions to assure timely publication of this book. I am indebted to these three wonderful and professional ladies for their untiring efforts on my behalf.

Finally, as the bedrock of this acknowledgment, the dedication, enthusiasm, attentiveness, and mostly cheerful attitude of our secretarial assistants, Sandra Sundve and Kathy Norred requires particular acclaim. In addition to all of the usual tasks attendant with a major manuscript revision, the final manuscript was prepared on computer using a unique software compatible with a sophisticated typesetting system. This nontrivial, occasionally severely frustrating process was successfully accomplished with great good grace by Ms. Sundve and Ms. Norred. We are proud to acknowledge publicly our very deep personal and professional appreciation of the magnificent work performed by these wonderful ladies.

John Henry, Jr. M.D., D.Sc.

Contents

Chapter 1

The Normal Cervical Spine

CHILD

The anatomy of the cervical spine of infants and children that has particular significance for the radiologist relates to ossification of the atlas and axis and hypermobility due to ligamentous laxity, especially the "pseudodislocation" at the C_2–C_3 and the C_3–C_4 levels (1).

Ossification of the atlas begins with the lateral masses during intrauterine life. At birth, however, neither the anterior nor the posterior arches are fused. During the second year, a center for the posterior tubercle appears and by the end of the fourth year, the posterior arch becomes completely fused. The anterior arch may fuse from a single center representing the anterior tubercle, from multiple centers on each side of the tubercle, or by direct extension from the lateral masses. Fusion is usually complete by the seventh to the tenth year.

The axis arises from five or six separate ossification centers depending upon whether the centrum has one or two centers (Fig. 1.1). The body of the axis is ossified at birth, but the posterior arches are only partially ossified. They fuse, posteriorly, by the second or third year and unite with the body by the seventh year.

The dens ossifies from two vertically oriented centers that fuse by the seventh fetal month. Cranially, a central cleft separates the tips of these ossification centers (Fig. 1.2). The ossiculum terminale, the ossification center for the tip of the dens (Fig. 1.3), may be radiographically visible. The os terminale usually unites with the body of the dens by age 11 or 12 years. Failure of the os terminale either to develop or unite with the dens may result in a bulbous, cleft dens tip (Fig. 1.4).

The dens is separated from the lateral masses by the neurocentral synchondroses and from the centrum by the subdental ("subchondral") synchondrosis (Fig. 1.1) all of which fuse between the third and sixth years. The neurocentral synchondrosis of the axis is not visible in the lateral radiograph because it is obscured by the density of the neural arch centers. However, it may be visible in frontal projection (Fig. 1.2).

1

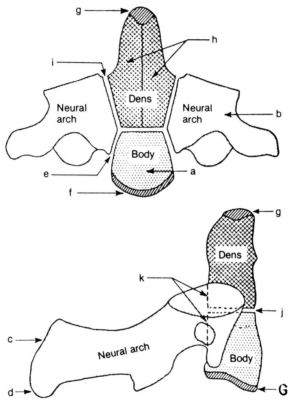

Figure 1.1. Schematic representation of ossification of the axis. Fusion of the neural arches, posteriorly, (*c*) usually occurs between the second and third years of life. The nuerocentral synchondrosis (*e*), the synchondrosis between the dens and the neural arches (*i*), and the subdental (subchondral) synchondrosis (*j*) all fuse between the third and sixth years. The ossification center for the tip of the dens is indicated by (*g*), the bifid tip of the spinous process by (*d*), the posterior surface of the dens and body by (*k*) and the inferior epiphyseal ring by (*f*). (From Bailey, D.K.: Normal cervical spine in infants and children. *Radiology* 59:713–714, 1952.)

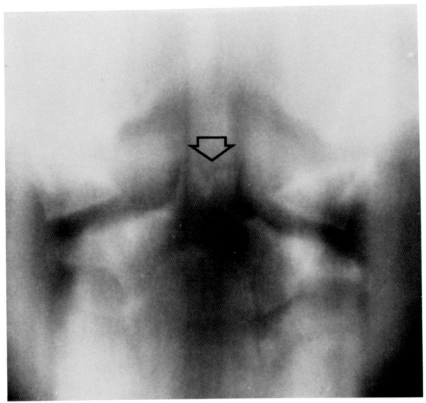

Figure 1.2. Normal appearance of the dens in a young child demonstrating the cleft between the tips of the ossification centers for the body of the dens (*arrow*).

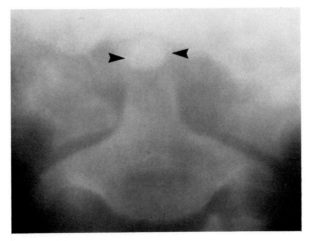

Figure 1.3. Ossiculum terminale (*arrowheads*).

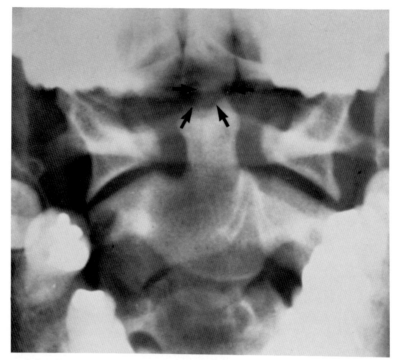

Figure 1.4. Anomalous, bulbous tip of the dens associated with a faintly visible ununited ossiculum terminale (*arrows*) in an adult.

The subdental (subchondral) synchondrosis is clearly visible as a transverse lucent defect separating the axis centrum from the base of the dens in the lateral radiograph (Figs. 1.5). It gradually decreases in width, but may persist as a thin radiolucent stripe with densely sclerotic margins until adolescence. As such, the synchondrosis may simulate a fracture (Fig. 1.6).

The "cervicocranium" includes the base of the skull, the atlas, the axis, and the second intervertebral disk (2,3,119,144,167). In infants and young children, normal laxity of the soft tissues of the cervicocranium may result in perplexing shadows on the lateral radigraph of the cervical spine.

Physiologic laxity of the retropharyngeal prevertebral soft tissues may simulate a retropharyngeal tumor, abscess, or hematoma unless great care is taken to obtain the lateral radiograph of the neck during maximum inspiration (Fig. 1.7) and, if neither clinically nor radiographically contraindicated, in extension.

Physiologic ligamentous laxity permits a greater range of motion at the atlantoaxial level during flexion and extension in infants and children than in adults. The anterior atlantodental interval (AADI), because of the looseness of the capsules and ligaments, may range from 2 to 5 mm with the maximum width occurring in flexion (4) (Fig.

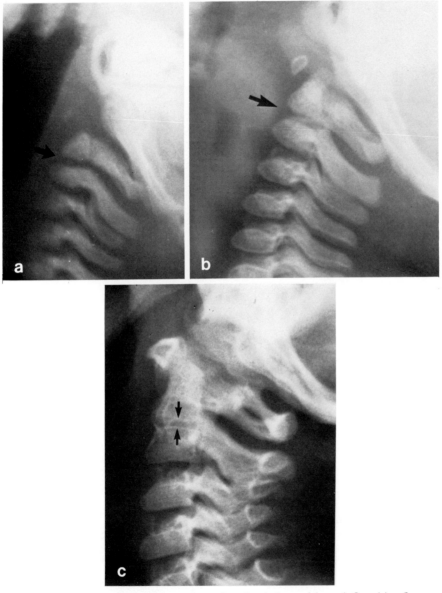

Figure 1.5.   Subchondral (subdental) synchondrosis (*arrows*) in an infant (*a*), a 3-year-old child (*b*), and a 6-year-old child (*c*).

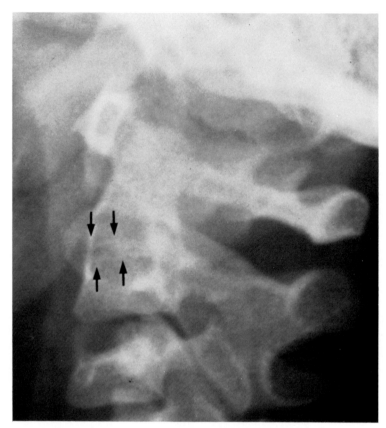

Figure 1.6. The "scar" of the fused subdental synchondrosis in an adult appears as two thin, parallel sclerotic lines (*arrows*) that should not be mistaken for a low (type III) dens fracture.

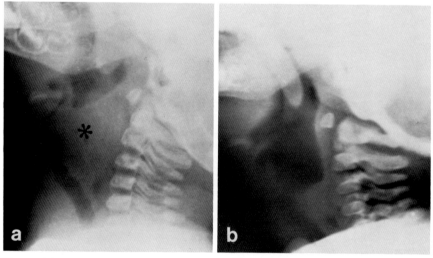

Figure 1.7. The effect of inspiration and positioning on the retropharyngeal soft tissues of an infant. (*a*) Exposure made during expiration and without cervical extension demonstrates a large retropharyngeal pseudomass (*). (*b*) Same patient, minutes later. Radiograph obtained during inspiration and with gentle cervical extension demonstrates normal prevertebral soft tissues and no mass.

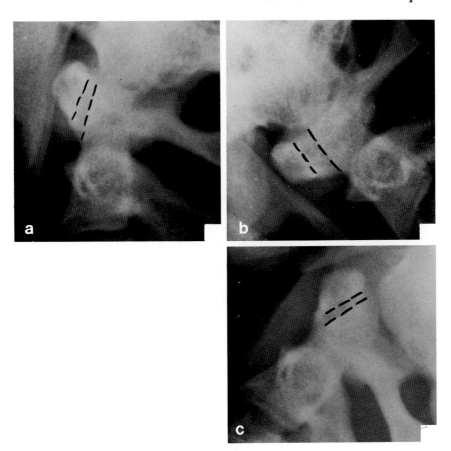

Figure 1.8. Neutral lateral (*a*), flexion (*b*), and extension (*c*) radiographs of the atlantoaxial articulation in a normal 5-year-old boy. The width of the space between the anterior arch of C_1 and the dens (AADI) measured 3 mm in neutral, 5 mm in flexion, and 2 mm in extension. Note, additionally, that the contiguous surfaces of the AADI are not parallel in flexion (*b*) or extension (*c*), further reflecting the physiologic movement of the atlas with respect to the axis.

1.8). The AADI, however, usually does not exceed 3 mm (5). In addition to change in width of the AADI in flexion and extension, its contiguous facets lose their parallelism.

Cattell and Filtzer (6) have noted that in 20% of normal children under 8 years of age, more than two-thirds of the anterior arch of the atlas lies above the tip of the dens in extension (Fig. 1.9).

"Pseudosubluxation" and "pseudodislocation" are terms applied to physiologic anterior displacement (translation) of C_2 or C_3 that is frequently seen in infants and young children. Physiologic anterior displacement of C_2 on C_3, and C_3 on C_4 occurs in 24% and 14%, respectively, of children to the age of 8 years (6). The mobility of these cervical segments has been attributed to the normal laxity of the ligaments of the cervical spine during childhood, to the shallow angle of incli-

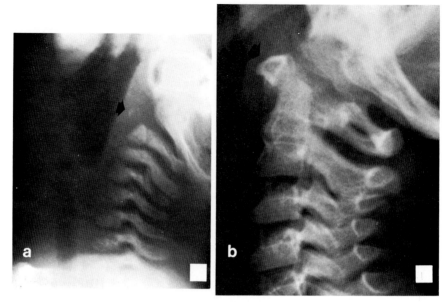

Figure 1.9.   Normal relationship of the anterior arch of the atlas (*arrow*) and the dens in extension. (*a*) Infant. (*b*) Young child. From Harris, J.H. Jr. & Harris, W.H.: *The Radiology of Emergency Medicine*. Baltimore, Williams & Wilkins, 1975.).

nation of the interfacetal joints at these levels, and to the fact that the C_2–C_3 level, which is the site of transition between the cervicocranium and the lower cervical spine, acts as the fulcrum for flexion and extension (6,7).

   In the child with a history of acute cervical spine trauma or of an accident that could have caused acute cervical spine injury, i.e., a motor vehicle or auto-pedestrian accident, or a fall from a height, the anterior position of a vertebra with respect to its subjacent member can represent a major diagnostic problem. The anterior position of the vertebra, alone, raises the possibility of significant cervical spine injury, such as unilateral interfacetal dislocation (UID), bilateral interfacetal dislocation (BID), traumatic spondylolisthesis, or hyperextension fracture-dislocation. The solution to the diagnostic problem rests with a detailed analysis of the involved segments for the presence of other radiographic signs of UID, BID, the posterior arch fractures of traumatic spondylolisthesis, or the posterior element fracture and/or dislocation of hyperextension fracture-dislocation. In the absence of any other signs of injury, resolution of the forward displacement rests with demonstration of a normal anatomic relationship of the posterior laminal lines of C_1 through C_3. Caffey (7) and Swischuk (8,9) have described the "posterior cervical line" (Fig. 1.10) and its relationship to the posterior laminar line of C_2 as indicating whether displacement of C_2 is physiologic or due to traumatic spondylolisthesis of C_2.

The posterior cervical line is an imaginary line extending from the posterior laminar line of the atlas to the posterior laminar line of C_3. Normally, in the neutral lateral radiograph of the cervical spine of a child, the posterior laminal line of C_2 lies upon, or 1 mm anterior or posterior to the imaginary posterior spinal line (Fig. 1.11). With an intact axis vertebra, the entire vertebra moves as a unit and, in flexion, the body of C_2 glides further anterior with respect to that of C_3 and the posterior laminal line of C_2 moves 1 to 3 mm anterior to the posterior spinal line. In extension, the intact axis translates posteriorly and its posterior laminal line may be 1 to 3 mm posterior to the posterior spinal line. The observation that the relationship of the axis body to the body of C_3 in neutral, flexion, and extension is the same as the relationship of the posterior laminal line of C_2 to the imaginary posterior spinal line, indicates that the axis vertebra is intact, thereby specifically excluding the diagnosis of traumatic spondylolisthesis (the hangman's fracture).

Traumatic spondylolisthesis, although common in adults, is rare in children. Flexion and extension lateral radiographs are not only unnecessary to establish the diagnosis of traumatic spondylolisthesis, but are frankly contraindicated. However, for the purpose of this discussion alone, if flexion and extension views were to be obtained in a child with a hangman's fracture, the axis body would be expected to translate anteriorly in flexion and posteriorly in extension. At the same time, the posterior laminal line of the separated posterior arch of the axis would maintain its normal relationship to the posterior spinal line by virtue of the intact posterior ligaments.

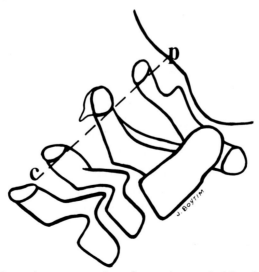

Figure 1.10.   Schematic representation of posterior cervical line (*pc*).

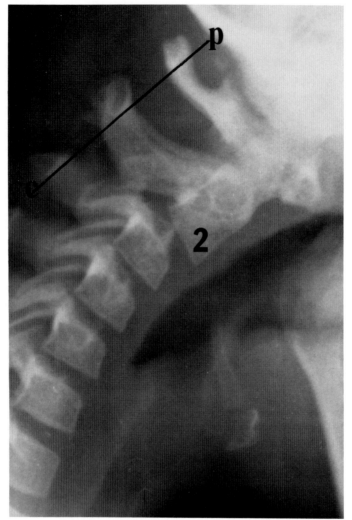

Figure 1.11. Pseudosubluxation of C₂ on C₃. The posterior laminal line of C₂ touches the posterior cervical line (*pc*).

ADULT

Cervicocranium

The anatomy of the cervical spine begins with the occiput and the occipital condyles. The occiput, the atlas, and the axis, when considered as a unit, are referred to as the "cervicocranium" (2,3). This designation is warranted by the distinctive morphology and physiology of this region that clearly differ from those of the lower cervical spine, which extends from C_3 through C_7. The effects of trauma to the cervicocranium are modified by its own unique structural characteristics.

    The atlanto-occipital joints are formed by the convex articulating surface of the occipital condyles and the concave superior facets of the lateral masses of the atlas.

The ligaments of the cervicocranium are important in maintaining stability throughout this region, are directly involved in the ranges of motion of the cervicocranium, and, anteriorly, contribute to the prevertebral soft tissue shadow on the lateral cervical radiograph.

The principle ligaments are (*a*) the dense anterior atlanto-occipital ligament (membrane) that extends from the superior surface of the anterior arch of the atlas to the anterior margin of the foramen magnum; (*b*) the dense alar ("check") ligaments which extend from the superolateral aspect of the tip of the dens to the occipital condyles and limit rotation of the cranium with respect to the atlas; (*c*) the transverse atlantal ligament that arches across the ring of the atlas, maintaining the relationship of the dens to the anterior arch of the atlas and, consequently, the normal width of the anterior atlantodental interval; and (*d*) the tectorial membrane, a strong dense band fixed to the dorsal surface of the axis that passes posterior to the transverse atlantal ligament of the dens and attaches to the occipital bone anterior to the foramen magnum. For practical purposes, the tectorial membrane may be considered the cranial extension of the posterior longitudinal ligament (10).

Lesser ligaments of this region include the apical dental ligament, a thin fibrous cord extending from the tip of the dens to the anterior margin of the foramen magnum (basion); the accessory ligaments that extend from the body of the dens near its base to each lateral mass of the atlas; the articular capsules; and the anterior and posterior atlantoaxial ligaments (Figs. 1.12 to 1.14).

The first cervical segment, the atlas (Fig. 1.14), is a unique ring-like vertebra characterized by the absence of a vertebral body. It consists of an anterior arch, a lateral mass on each side, and a posterior arch. It does not contain pedicles or laminae, as do other cervical vertebrae, and has no true spinous process. The anterior and posterior arches are relatively thin. The lateral masses, on the other hand, are heavy, thick structures. Each has a concave superior and a convex inferior articulating surface. A rudimentary transverse process extends laterally from each mass and contains the transverse foramen through which passes the vertebral artery.

The short, dense, thick transverse atlantal ligament extends between the medial surfaces of the lateral masses (Figs. 1.13 and 1.14) and maintains the normal relationship of the dens to the anterior arch of C_1.

The second cervical vertebra, the axis, is the largest and heaviest cervical segment (Fig. 1.15). Like the remainder of the cervical vertebrae, it consists of a body, bilateral masses (articular masses, "pillars"),

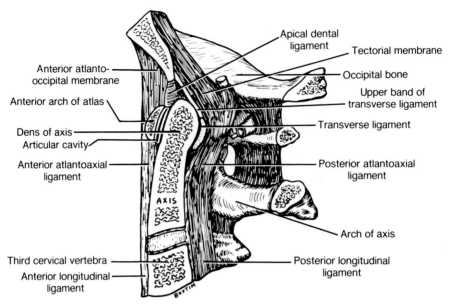

Figure 1.12. Schematic sagittal representation of the cervicocranium. (From Harris, J. H. Jr. & Harris, W. H.: *The Radiology of Emergency Medicine.* Baltimore, Williams & Wilkins, 1975.)

laminae, and a thick, heavy, spinous proccess. It is unique by virtue of the odontoid process (dens), an upward extension of the body of the axis that serves as the pivotal point of atlantal rotation. The superior articulating facets of the axis are convex, while the inferior facets face obliquely forward and downward.

The atlas and axis articulate through four joints, the median and the bilateral atlantoaxial joints (11). The articulation between the pos-

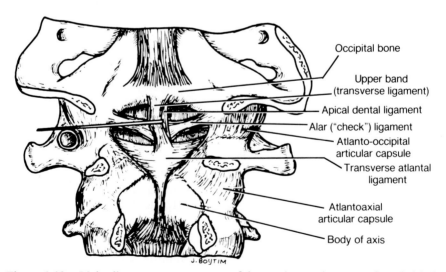

Figure 1.13. Major ligamentous structures of the cervicocranium, seen from behind.

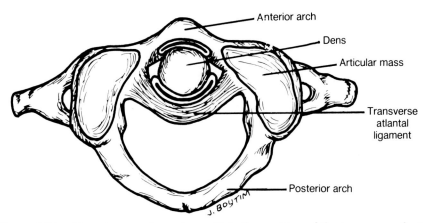

Figure 1.14. The atlas seen from above. Note the position of the transverse atlantal ligament to the dens.

terior surface of the anterior arch of C_1 and the anterior surface of the dens and that between the posterior surface of the dens and the transverse atlantal ligament together constitute the median atlantoaxial (pivot) joint. Each of these components has a true, separate, synovial joint space (Figs. 1.12 and 1.14).

The lateral atlantoaxial joints are formed by the contiguous articulating surfaces of the lateral masses of the atlas and axis. These joints are arthrodial, and each articulating surface of each joint is somewhat convex. In the neutral position, therefore, the articulating surfaces of the atlas and axis are in contact only at the highest points of their convex surfaces. During rotation, the inferior facets of the atlas, moving

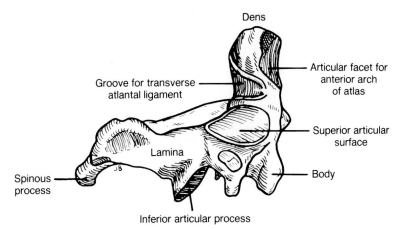

Figure 1.15. The axis seen in lateral projection. Note that the convex superior facet is horizontally situated while the inferior facet is obliquely anteriorly and inferiorly oriented to form the superior component of the highest interfacetal joint. (From Harris, J.H. Jr. & Harris, W.H.: *The Radiology of Emergency Medicine.* Baltimore, Williams & Wilkins, 1975.)

either anteriorly or posteriorly, come to be in contact with the superior facet of the axis at some point lower than the apex of its convex surface. This has been referred to as "telescoping" (12) and is the explanation for "vertical approximation," the term used by Hohl (13) to describe the apparent decrease in combined vertical height of the atlas and axis in extreme rotation.

The roentgen appearance of the atlantoaxial articulation in frontal projection, i.e., the "open-mouth" view, is seen in Figure 1.16. The important observations are that (*a*) the atlas sits squarely upon the axis with the dens symmetrically situated between the lateral masses of the atlas, (*b*) the lateral atlantoaxial joint spaces are open and their contiguous surfaces are parallel, (*c*) the lateral margins of the contiguous facets of the atlas and axis are on essentially the same vertical plane and are symmetrical, and (*d*) that the bifid spinous process of the axis is in the midline.

The physiologic motions of rotation and lateral tilt produce radiographically discernible changes in the relationship of the atlas and axis that must be recognized and understood. Since the mechanism of injury of atlantoaxial rotary displacement ("torticollis") and fixation

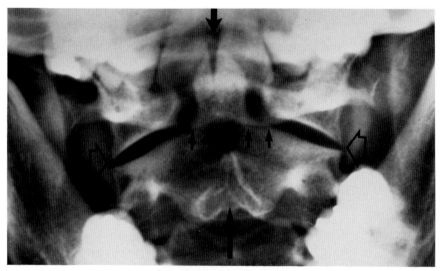

Figure 1.16.   The atlantoaxial articulation seen in the open-mouth view. The dens is centrally located between the lateral masses of the axis, the lateral margins of the lateral atlantoaxial joints are symmetrical and are on essentially the same vertical plane (*open arrows*), and the spinous process of C$_2$ (*long arrow at bottom of figure*) is in the midline. Two frequently perplexing natural artifacts are illustrated. The space between the central maxillary incisor teeth (*large arrow at top of figure*) could be misinterpreted as a vertical defect of the dens. The thin, curvilinear, transverse lucent band at the base of the dens (*small arrows*) is caused by the Mach effect of the superimposed inferior margin of the posterior arch of the atlas. This may be mistaken for a fracture line. (From Harris, J.H. Jr.: Acute injuries of the spine. *Semin. Roentgenol.* 13:53, 1978.)

and of acute traumatic atlantoaxial rotary dislocation is a combination of rotation and lateral tilt of C_1 on C_2, the radiographic signs of each of these conditions, as well as those of physiologic rotation and tilt, are identical and their distinction must, therefore, be made on clinical grounds.

Fielding (12) has shown, cineradiographically, that during rotation of the head, the skull and atlas turn as a unit with the atlas pivoting on the axis, about the dens. Simply stated, C_1 rotates on C_2. During rotation, the following physiologic changes in the relationship of the lateral masses of the atlas and axis occur: (*a*) As the head rotates in one direction, the contralateral lateral mass of the atlas rotates forward and medially, becoming rectangular in appearance. The distance between this lateral mass and the dens decreases, and the medial and lateral margins of the inferior facet of the atlas lie medial to their counterparts of the axis. (*b*) The lateral mass of the atlas on the side of the direction of the rotation moves posteriorly and becomes truncated in configuration. The distance between this lateral mass of the atlas and the dens remains unaltered or decreases slightly, and the margins of the articular facets become asymmetrical (Figs. 1.17 and 1.18).

As rotation increases toward maximum, the convex inferior articulating facets of the atlas rotate off the convex superior facets of the axis. Whereas in neutral position these facets are in apposition at the highest point of their convex surfaces and an open joint space is clearly evident (Fig. 1.16), with rotation the high point of the inferior facet of the atlas drops below the high point of the superior facet of the axis and the lateral atlantoaxial joint spaces become narrow or obliterated in direct proportion to the amount of rotation. When the atlas rotates off the high point of the convex articulating surfaces of the axis, the total vertical height of the atlantoaxial complex decreases (Fig. 1.19), i.e., "telescoping" (12) or "vertical approximation." (13).

Another physiologic effect that occurs with increasing rotation relates to the axis. During the early phase of the rotational range, the axis remains stationary. With further rotation of the head, the axis rotates in the same direction and its bifid spinous process deviates away from the midline in the opposite direction (Fig. 1.19).

Lateral tilt or bending is simply allowing the head to deviate off the midline to one side or the other. For the purposes of definition and demonstration, lateral tilt will be assumed to be a pure motion completely devoid of any rotational component. (Pure lateral tilt is difficult to accomplish and probably occurs naturally only rarely.)

During lateral tilt, the skull and atlas move as a unit and glide from the midline toward the side of the tilt. For example, if the head is tilted to the left, the atlas glides to the left with respect to the axis. Consequently, the space between the right lateral mass and the dens

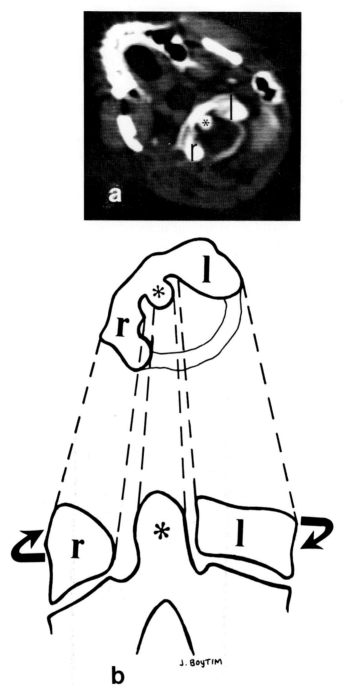

Figure 1.17. CT scan of the normal atlantoaxial articulation made with the head rotated to the right (*a*). The line drawing (*b*) depicts the relation of the atlas and axis as seen on an "open-mouth" radiograph obtained with the patient in the same position as the CT scan. The left lateral mass of the atlas (*l*) has rotated anteriorly and the right lateral mass (*r*) posteriorly. The anteriorly rotated lateral mass presents a greater transverse dimension to the x-ray beam and appears increased transversely in the open-mouth projection. The space between this lateral mass and the dens decreases. Conversely, the opposite lateral mass assumes a truncated configuration and its lateral atlantodental interval either increases or maintains normal width.

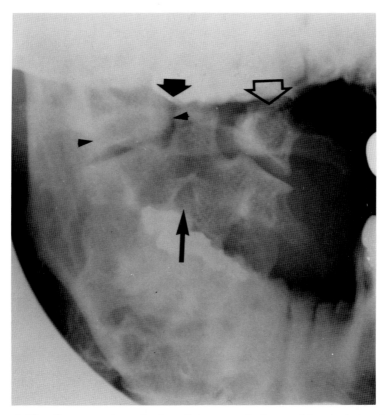

Figure 1.18. Open-mouth projection of the normal atlantoaxial articulation during moderate rotation to the left. The right lateral mass of the atlas has rotated anteriorly and appears to have increased in transverse diameter (*small arrowheads*). The distance between this lateral mass and the dens is narrowed (*solid arrow*), and the margins of its articulating facet lie medial to those of the superior facet of the axis. The left lateral mass of the atlas (*open arrow*) has rotated posteriorly and is truncated in configuration. The margins of the left lateral atlantoaxial joint are asymmetrical. The spinous process of the axis (*long arrow*) remains in the midline.

decreases while the space between the dens and the left lateral mass of the axis increases slightly. The margins of the contiguous articular facets of the atlas and axis become similarly asymmetrical (Fig. 1.20).

The axis and the subjacent vertebrae rotate during lateral tilt. This normal, physiologic component of lateral bending (tilt) occurs early during lateral bending, and the rotation is in the direction of the tilt. For example, if the head is tilted to the left, the axis rotates to the left, causing the bifid spinous process of the axis to deviate to the right of the midline. It may be surprising to learn that the rotation of the axis occurs earlier in lateral bending than during rotation. However, this fact has been conclusively demonstrated by Fielding (12) and is illustrated in Figure 1.21. The importance of this physiologic fact will become evident in the discussion of atlantoaxial injury.

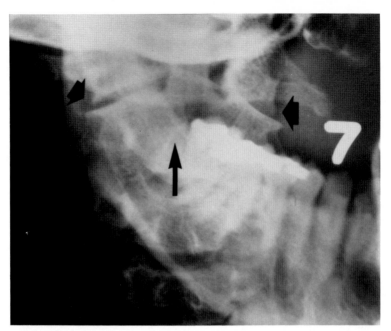

Figure 1.19. Normal atlantoaxial articulation in marked rotation. Narrowing and obliteration of the lateral joint spaces due to vertical approximation are indicated by the solid arrows. The asymmetry of the margins of these joints is physiologic. The spinous process of the axis (*long arrow*) is deviated to the right of the midline, indicating rotation of the axis in the same direction as the rotation of the head.

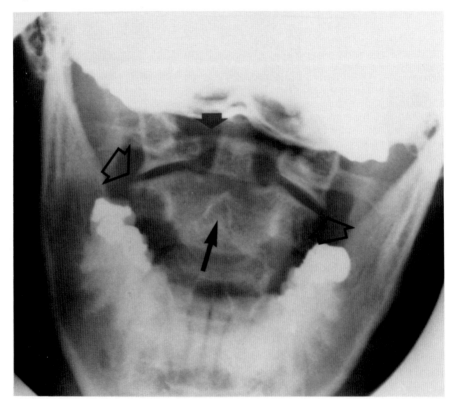

Figure 1.20. Normal atlantoaxial articulation in minimal lateral tilt to the left. The atlas has glided to the left. The space between the right lateral mass of the atlas and the dens has decreased (*solid arrow*) while that on the left has widened. The lateral margins of the lateral atlantoaxial joint spaces are physiologically asymmetrical (*open arrows*). At this minimal degree of tilt, the axis has not rotated and its spinous process (*long arrow*) remains in the midline.

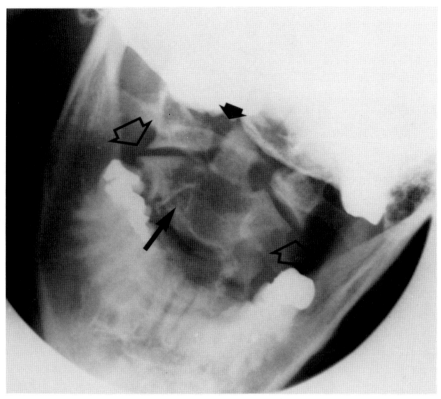

Figure 1.21. Normal atlantoaxial articulation in moderate lateral tilt to the left. The physiologic changes illustrated in Figure 1.20 are accentuated. In addition, with greater tilt, physiologic rotation of the axis to the left has resulted in its spinous process (*long arrow*) being deviated to the right of the midline.

The lateral radiographic appearance of the cervicocranium of a normal adult is seen in Figure 1.22. It is important to be aware that air in the pharynx outlines the soft palate and uvula, the base of the tongue and the naso-oropharyngeal airway. The shadow representing the normal soft tissue structures of the posterior wall of the naso-oropharynx is closely adherent to the anterior surface of the atlas and axis and extends superiorly to the clivus and inferiorly to become continuous with the soft tissues of the posterior wall of the hypopharynx. Above the level of the anterior arch of the atlas, this soft tissue shadow represents principally the anterior atlanto-occipital ligament and from the anterior inferior corner of the axis to the atlas, principally the anterior atlantoaxial ligament, which is, in effect, the cephalic extension of the anterior longitudinal ligament.

Adenoidal tissue, commonly present in the nasopharynx, produces a homogeneous, smoothly lobulated mass of varying size and configuration (Figs. 1.23 and 1.24). In the lateral radiograph of the face or cervical spine, the surface of the adenoidal tissue is demarcated by air

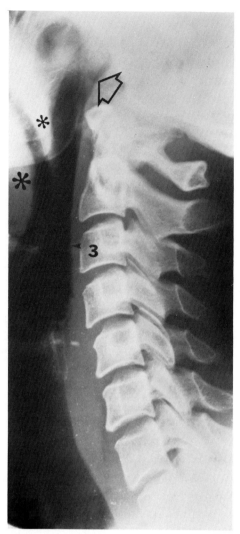

Figure 1.22. Soft tissues of the naso-orohypopharynx of a normal adult. The posterior wall of the nasopharynx is indicated by the *open arrow*, the soft palate and uvula by the *small asterisk* and the base of the tongue by the *large asterisk*. The *arrowhead* indicates the normal appearance of the prevertebral soft tissues anterior to the body of C$_3$ on the 6-foot lateral radiograph of an adult cervical spine. At this level, the soft tissue shadow should not normally exceed 4 mm with a target-film distance of 6 feet and the air-soft tissue interface should be sharply defined.

inferiorly and anteriorly. The latter observation distinguishes this physiologic mass from the nasopharyngeal hematoma commonly associated with major midface fractures (Fig. 1.25).

The normal relationship between the posterior surface of the anterior arch of the atlas and the anterior surface of the dens (anterior atlanto-dental interval, AADI) is maintained by the transverse atlantal ligament. Assuming a target-film distance of 6 feet, the AADI does not

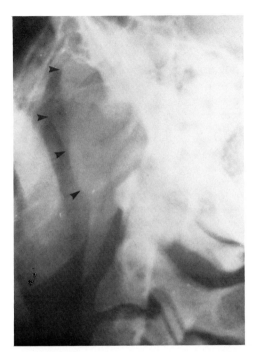

Figure 1.23. The smoothly lobulated soft tissue mass (*arrowheads*) high in the naso-pharynx is typical of adenoidal tissue. Air outlining the anterior surface of the mass distinguishes it from a pharyngeal hematoma associated with a midface fracture. The abrupt angulation at the junction of the mass and the normal cervicocranial prever-tebral soft tissue shadow is inconsistent with the mass representing a hematoma sec-ondary to an acute cervical cranial injury.

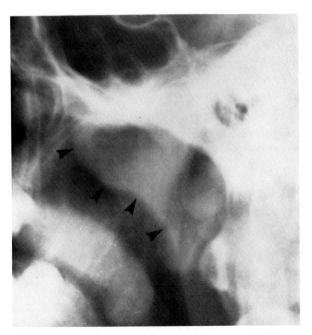

Figure 1.24. This adenoidal mass (*arrowheads*) in a young adult has many of the dis-tinguishing characteristics described in Figure 1.23.

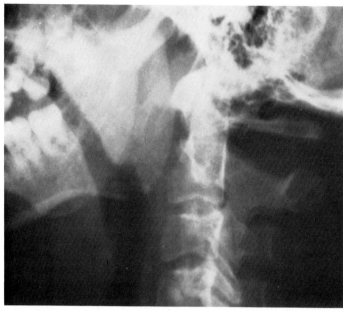

Figure 1.25. The soft tissue density that completely fills the nasopharynx, which is inseparable from the facial skeleton and the nasal surface of the soft palate and uvula and which extends to the posterior pharyngeal wall, represents a hematoma associated with a LeFort III midface fracture. Compare this soft tissue mass with that of adenoidal tissue in Figures 1.23 and 1.24.

normally exceed 3 mm in adults in lateral neutral, flexion, and extension radiographs (Fig. 1.26).

The posterior arch of the atlas is small compared to the size of the occiput and the heavy spinous process of the axis. In a properly positioned lateral radiograph, each half of the posterior arch of C_1 should be superimposed upon the other half with a distinct soft tissue space between the posterior ring of C_1 and the occiput above and the laminae and spinous process of the axis below. The width of these spaces, especially the occipitoatlantal space, normally varies with flexion and extension (Fig. 1.26).

Lower Cervical Vertebrae

The third through the seventh cervical vertebrae are uniform in configuration but increase gradually in size, with the seventh being the largest and heaviest. Each vertebra consists of a body, paired pedicles, articular masses, laminae, and a single spinous process. A transverse process projects laterally from the superolateral aspect of each side of the vertebral body and fuses distally and posteriorly with the anterior surface of the articular mass. The transverse process contains the foramen transversarium through which passes the vertebral artery (Fig. 1.27).

The vertebral body is bounded superiorly and inferiorly by its end-plates which are adherent to the adjacent intervertebral disk. The cephalad projection of the lateral aspect of the superior end-plate is the uncinate process, which, together with the contiguous lateral margin of the immediately superior vertebra, forms the joint of Luschka.

The articular masses ("pillar") are dense, heavy, rhomboid-shaped structures bounded superiorly and inferiorly by their smooth articulating facets. The posterolateral cortex of the articular mass is a curved surface that is convex posterolaterally. An arc of this surface which, in lateral projection, is tangent to the x-ray beam produces a distinct, vertically oriented, posteriorly convex radiographic "line" on the lateral radiograph, which is referred to as the posterior cortex of the articular mass (Fig. 1.28). Because this "line" connects the posterior margins of the superior and inferior articulating facets, it helps to

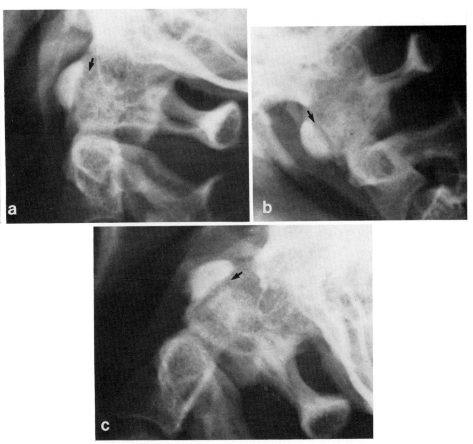

Figure 1.26. The normal, constant relationship between the anterior arch of the atlas and the anterior cortex of the dens (the anterior atlantodental interval (*arrow*)) is maintained in adults by the transverse atlantal ligament in neutral (*a*), flexed (*b*), and extended (*c*) positions.

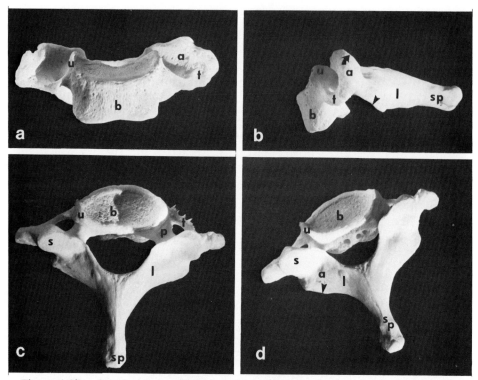

Figure 1.27. A typical lower (C_3–C_7) vertebra from frontal (*a*), lateral (*b*), superior (*c*), and superolateral oblique (*d*) perspectives. Wherever seen, *b* is the vertebral body; *t*, the transverse process including the foramen transversarium; *p*, pedicle; *a* articular mass; *s* and *curved arrow*, superior facet; *arrowhead*, inferior facet; *l*, lamina; *sp*, spinous process; and *u*, the uncinate process.

identify the articular masses and the relationship of the "line" to its opposite counterpart serves as one of the indicators of cervical spine rotation.

The paired laminae are direct posteromedial extensions of the articular masses. Each lamina lies above and slightly posterior to its subjacent lamina (Fig. 1.27). The laminae form the posterolateral aspect of the spinal canal and fuse posteriorly to form the base of the spinous process, which is a midline structure. The thin vertical strip of internal laminar cortex at the base of the spinous process which is tangent to the x-ray beam in lateral projection forms another important radiographic "line," the posterior laminal line (Fig. 1.28), which marks the posterior extent of the spinal canal.

The contiguous articulating facets of the lateral masses from C_2 through C_7 comprise the interfacetal (facetal, apophyseal) joints. The inferior facet of the vertebra above constitutes the superior facet of the joint and the superior articulating facet of the vertebra below constitutes the inferior facet of the joint. The inferior facet of the vertebra

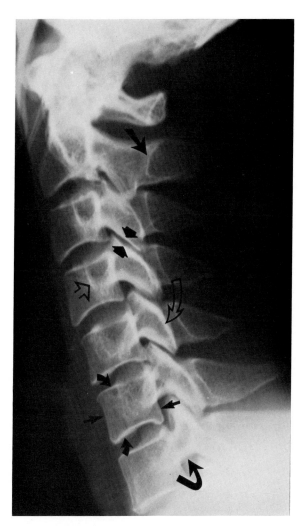

Figure 1.28. Lateral radiograph of a normal adult cervical spine in neutral position. From anterior to posterior, the anterior and posterior cortices of the vertebral body are indicated by *small arrows*, the superior and inferior end-plates by *curved arrows*, the transverse processes by the *open arrow*, the incompletely seen pedicles by the *reversed arrow*, the superior and inferior facets of an interfacetal joint by *arrowheads*, the posterior "cortex" of the articular mass by the *open curved arrow*, and the posterior laminal line by the *large oblique arrow*.

above is directed anteriorly and inferiorly, while the superior facet of the subjacent vertebra is oriented posteriorly and superiorly. The plane of the interfacetal joints is angled approximately 35° anteriorly from the vertical (Fig. 1.28). For purposes of clarity, consistency, and simplicity of expression, the articulating facets will, in all subsequent discussions, be defined as they comprise the interfacetal joints, i.e., the superior facet (of the joint) and the inferior facet (of the joint).

The superior facets are normally situated above and behind the inferior facets and the contiguous facets are normally parallel. The posterior margins of the articulating facets are closely parallel, symmetrical and, in the neutral position, at each level are on or very close to the same vertical plane (Fig. 1.28).

Soft tissue structures with less specific functions than those of the cervicocranium are present throughout the cervical area and are important to cervical stability and motion. The ligamentum nuchae extends deep into the neck and, attaching to the spinous process of the cervical segments, forms a septum between the muscles on each side of the posterior aspect of the neck. The supraspinous ligament (Fig. 1.29) is a strong fibrous component of the ligamentum nuchae that connects the apices of the spinous processes from the external occipital protuberance to the spinous process of C_7.

The interspinous ligaments (Fig. 1.29) are thin membranous structures that connect adjacent spinous processes. They extend from the base to the tip of each spinous process.

The thin, loose capsules of the interfacetal joints (Fig. 1.29) attach to the margins of the articular surfaces of the adjacent vertebrae.

The ligamenta flava (Fig. 1.30) are thick, dense, broad structures that connect the laminae of adjacent vertebrae. These ligaments arise from the ventral surface of the lamina above and pass inferiorly to attach to the dorsal surface of the lamina below where the laminae fuse to form the base of the spinous process.

The posterior longitudinal ligament (Fig. 1.29) extends from the axis to the sacrum. It is a dense broad ligament lying within the ventral

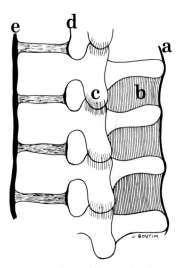

Figure 1.29.   Schematic representation of the major ligaments of the lower cervical spine. *a*, supraspinous ligament, *b*, the interspinous ligament; *c*, articular capsule of an interfacetal joint; *d*, posterior longitudinal ligament; *e*, anterior longitudinal ligament. (From Harris, J.H. Jr.: Acute injuries of the spine. *Semin. Roentgenol.* 13:53, 1978.)

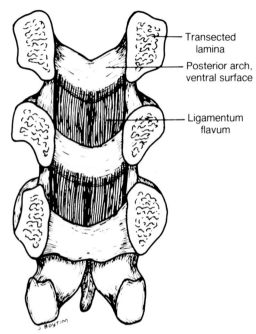

Transected lamina

Posterior arch, ventral surface

Ligamentum flavum

Figure 1.30. Schematic representation of the ventral aspect of the posterior neural arch. Note that the ligamenta flava arise from the ventral surface of the lamina above and insert on the posterior surface of the lamina below.

surface of the spinal canal, closely adherent to the posterior surface of the vertebral bodies and disks.

The intervertebral disks (Fig. 1.29), being interposed between contiguous surfaces of adjacent vertebrae, constitute the chief connection between the vertebral bodies. Their principle attachment to the vertebral end-plates is through the dense Sharpey's fibers (Fig. 8.31) which are a component of the annulus fibrosus and which play an important role in hyperextension dislocation. The intervertebral disks are closely adherent to the anterior and posterior longitudinal ligaments.

The dense, strong anterior longitudinal ligament (Fig. 1.29) extends from the anterior inferior surface of the axis (C_2) to the sacrum. It is closely adherent to the intervertebral disks and the adjacent prominent end-plate margins of the vertebrae, but is not tightly adherent to the concavity of the anterior surfaces of the vertebral bodies.

The anteroposterior radiograph of the cervical spine of a normal adult is seen in Figure 1.31. Because of the density caused by superimposition of the mandible and occiput, the atlantoaxial articulation is usually not seen in the frontal projection; however, the lower five cervical and the upper thoracic segments are usually included. The

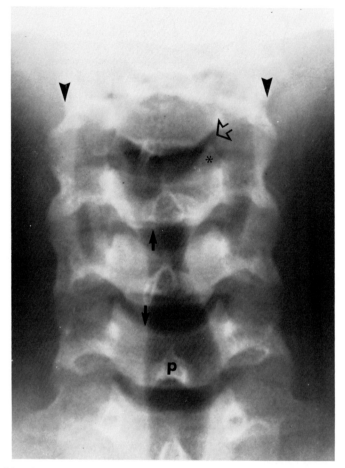

Figure 1.31. Anteroposterior radiograph of the lower cervical spine of a nontrauma adult patient. The superior and inferior end-plates are indicated by *arrows*, the uncinate process by an *asterisk*, and the joint of Luschka by the *open arrow*. The spinous processes (*p*) are in the midline. The smoothly undulating cortical "margin" of the lateral columns are indicated by *arrowheads*.

superior and inferior end-plates, the lateral cortical margins, and the uncinate processes of the vertebral bodies, as well as the joints of Luschka are usually clearly seen in this projection.

The interfacetal joint spaces, which are angled approximately 35° posteroinferiorly, are not normally visualized because of the super-imposition of the articular masses. As a result of the superimposition, the lateral cortical margins of the articular masses appear, in antero-posterior projection, as a seemingly continuous, smoothly undulating, sharply defined density at the lateral edges of the cervical spine, giving the appearance of a solid column of bone, i.e., the "lateral column." Alterations in the appearance of this radiographic optical illusion are very helpful in the recognition of posterior column injuries such as

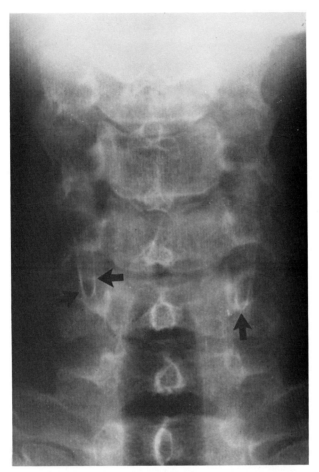

Figure 1.32.   Calcified thyroid cartilage (*arrows*).

may occur with distraction during flexion or with compression during hyperextension. The spinous processes are in the midline.

The margins of the air shadow in the upper trachea and subglottic area are tapered symmetrically toward the midline. When calcified, the lateral walls of the thyroid cartilage may cast thin, double, parallel, lineal densities approximately 3 mm apart on each side of the neck (Fig. 1.32). These should not be mistaken for either an opaque foreign body or a fracture fragment.

In contradistinction to the frontal radiograph, the lateral projection of the cervical spine (Fig. 1.33) should include the atlas, axis, and the skull base. The vertebral bodies are normally nearly square or slightly rectangular in the anteroposterior dimension. The contiguous surfaces of the disk spaces, which are normally parallel, may be modified by anomalies of the cervical vertebrae or by localized or diffuse osteoarthritis. The transverse processes are superimposed upon the

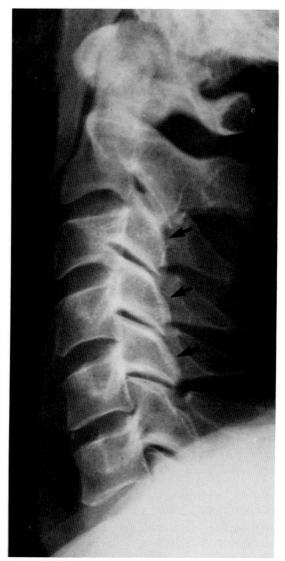

Figure 1.33.   Lateral radiograph of a normal adult cervical spine. The vertebrae are aligned in a gentle lordotic configuration. The posterior margins of the vertebral bodies constitute a continuous concave sweep, while the curve of the anterior surface is convex. The lateral (articular) masses are superimposed and so, consequently, are the interfacetal joint spaces and their superior and inferior articulating facets. The paired posterior cortical surfaces of the lateral masses (*arrows*) are superimposed and appear as a single cortical density.

vertebral bodies and pedicles and appear as complete or incomplete broad "U"-shaped densities with double or wide indistinct margins. The pedicles are not visualized in lateral projection because of their shortness, their posterolateral oblique orientation, and the density of the superimposed articular masses and transverse processes.

Positioning for the lateral radiograph is critical in order to assure, as nearly as is possible, a true lateral examination (Fig. 1.33). The criteria used to evaluate the accuracy of positioning pertain to the paired posterior structures and not the vertebral bodies, which will be nearly square or slightly rectangular regardless of even moderate degrees of rotation. In a true lateral radiograph of the cervical spine, the lateral masses should be so precisely superimposed that, even though they are paired structures, they appear as one with a single posterior cortical line. The articulating surfaces (facets) of the interfacetal joints should be superimposed so that it appears as though there is a single interfacetal joint space at each level. The posterior margins of the articulating facets of the apophyseal joints should be closely superimposed.

From the level of the third spinous process downward, the interspinous spaces are of approximately the same height, although they may vary considerably depending upon the size or shape of the spinous processes. The second interspinous space is commonly greater than the others. The laminae, however, are consistently much more uniform in size and, consequently, the interlaminar spaces are consistently of more uniform height (Fig. 1.33). Therefore, an increase in height of an interlaminar space in a patient with a history of cervical spine injury is a sensitive and reliable sign of posterior ligament complex tear such as occurs in anterior subluxation (hyperflexion sprain) (Figs. 4.6 to 4.8).

Even slight rotation causes anterior displacement of the articular masses of one side with respect to those of the opposite side. Radiographically, this is evident by the lack of superimposition of the posterior cortical margins of the articular masses and of the interfacetal joints. If the entire spine is rotated uniformly, i.e., if the patient is not in a true lateral position, the amount of asymmetry of the posterior cortices of the lateral masses will be uniform throughout the cervical area (Fig. 1.34). Improper positioning for the lateral cervical spine radiograph caused only by rotation of the head with the patient in true lateral position is characterized by gradually increasing amounts of asymmetry of the lateral masses from the lower to the upper cervical segments (Fig. 1.35).

It is important to be aware of the effect of these two forms of improper positioning upon the lateral radiograph of the cervical spine so that these positional changes are not misinterpreted (Fig. 1.36) as the rotational component of unilateral interfacetal dislocation.

Assessment of the cervical prevertebral soft tissue shadow is an essential and integral part of the examination of the lateral radiograph of the cervical spine. In a patient with acute cervical spine trauma, prevertebral soft tissue swelling reflects edema and hemorrhage and may be the only, or the most obvious, radiographic sign of cervical

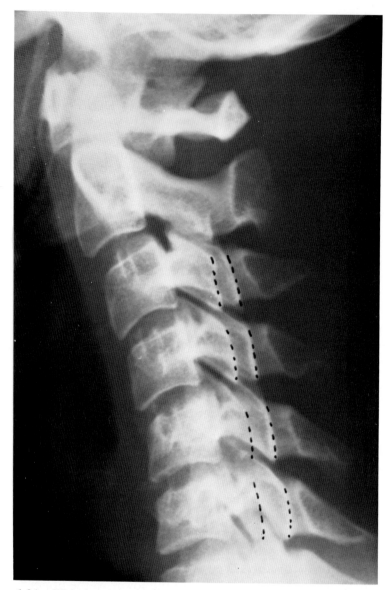

Figure 1.34. With the entire body rotated slightly forward on its central axis, the articular masses are no longer superimposed. The posterior cortical surfaces (*broken lines*) of one side lie anterior to those of the opposite side. The degree of lack of superimposition is similar at each level because the entire cervical spine has rotated as a unit.

injury. The width of the soft tissue shadow anterior to the body of C_3 is an extremely important landmark. Hay (14) has developed a formula by which the normal width of this soft tissue shadow can be calculated, based on patient age. A more practical and useful standard of the normal width of the cervical prevertebral soft tissues has been described

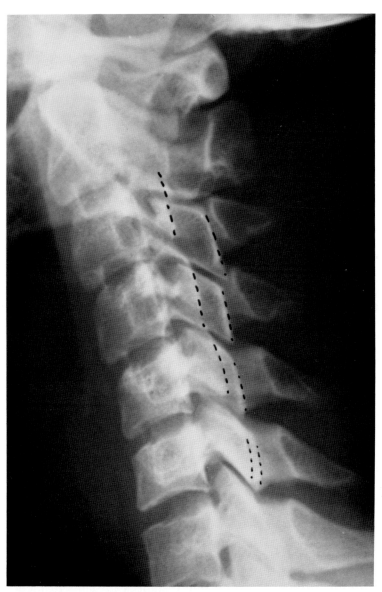

Figure 1.35. Improper positioning caused by rotation of the head alone. In this example, the body is in lateral position relative to its central axis, but the head has been allowed to rotate slightly. Because rotation of the head involves primarily the atlas and axis, there is progressively greater lack of superimposition of the articular masses from the lower through the upper segments.

by Weir (15), who determined that the normal width of the prevertebral soft tissue shadow anterior to the body of C_3, should not exceed 4 mm in an adult (Fig. 1.22), assuming a traget-film distance of 6 feet. Edeiken-Monroe et al. (16) have shown that with a target-film distance of 1 m (40 inches) the magnification factor is 0.4. Therefore, in lateral

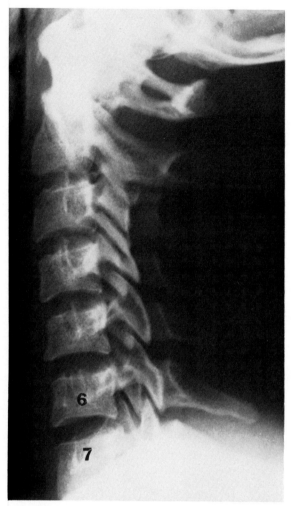

Figure 1.36.   Lateral radiograph of the cervical spine obtained in such an extreme degree of rotation that the position of the interfacetal joints at the C_6–C_7 level simulates unilateral interfacetal dislocation.

examinations of the cervical spine obtained with portable equipment or with units with fixed target-film distances (usually 40 inches), the thickness of the prevertebral soft tissues anterior to the body of C_3 in an adult may normally be as much as 7 mm. Another valuable characteristic of the cervical prevertebral soft tissues is that the air-soft tissue interface is normally sharp and distinct, rather than indistinct or irregular, as usually occurs with edema or hemorrhage.

Flexion and extension occur in a gradual, sequential fashion with the amount of motion being greatest at the upper levels (Fig. 1.37). Fielding (17) stated: "Below the second cervical vertebra, motion at one interspace gradually does not occur without similar motion taking place at other levels." During flexion, there is a continuum of movement from the lower through the upper segments, characterized by each successively higher segment translating (moving) progressively further forward while pivoting on its anterior inferior corner. This change in the relationship of adjacent vertebrae may occur in one of two ways, each of which has a distinctive radiographic appearance. In one instance, the forward translation of each successively higher segment may be smoothly continuous so that connecting the posterior cortical margins of the centra results in an uninterrupted anteriorly concave imaginary line (Fig. 1.38). In the other instance, flexion may occur as each successively higher segment translates anteriorly a discrete distance so that flexion occurs through a series of seemingly separate, disconnected, segmental anterior (forward) increments. On the lateral radiograph (Fig.1.37), the vertebral bodies appear to have moved as separate, discrete segments, simultaneously but independent of each other, to achieve flexion. The posterior cortical margin of each cervical vertebral body is offset from the adjacent segments by a distance that may normally be as much as 3 mm (18).

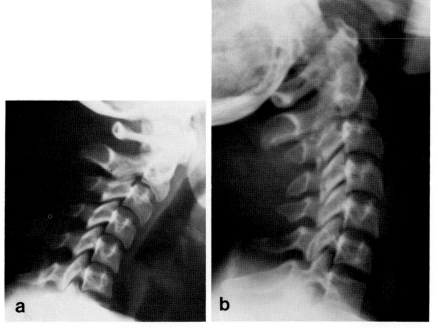

Figure 1.37.   Lateral radiograph of a normal adult cervical spine in flexion (*a*). Each successively higher segment pivots and glides slightly more forward than the segment below. Movement is greatest at the higher levels. This results in a uniform reversal of the normal cervical lordotic curve. All of the interspaces are narrowed anteriorly and widened posteriorly. The superior facets glide forward on the inferior facets and the interspinous spaces widen. In extension (*b*), all of the changes of flexion are reversed.

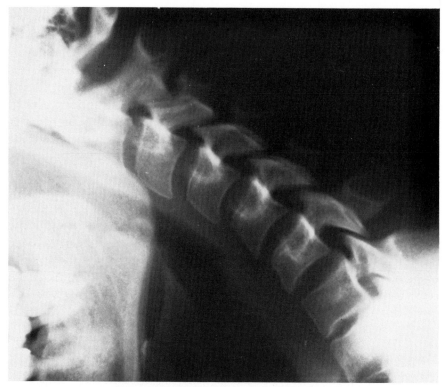

Figure 1.38.   In this flexion lateral radiograph, each successively higher segment has moved anteriorly a slightly greater distance than its subjacent vertebra. The amount of forward translation at each level is part of a craniocaudad continuum and an imaginary line connecting the posterior cortex of each segment is a smooth continuous anterior concave arc.

In extension, these movements are reversed and each successively higher segment may be posteriorly displaced with respect to the subjacent vertebra as much as 3 mm physiologically (Fig. 1.39).

The routine oblique radiograph of the cervical spine is made with the patient rotated approximately 45° off the frontal (or lateral) position. In positioning the patient for the oblique projection, it is important that the entire body be rotated about the longitudinal axis of the spine rather than simply rotating the head and neck. A properly positioned oblique radiograph of a normal adult spine is seen in Figure 1.40.

The purpose of the oblique projection is to visualize the pedicles, the intervertebral foramina, the articular masses, and their interfacetal joints, and the relationship of the laminae, which are posteromedial extensions of the articular masses, with respect to one another (Fig. 1.40). In a properly positioned oblique view, the central beam passes directly through the intervertebral foramina, clearly delineating the

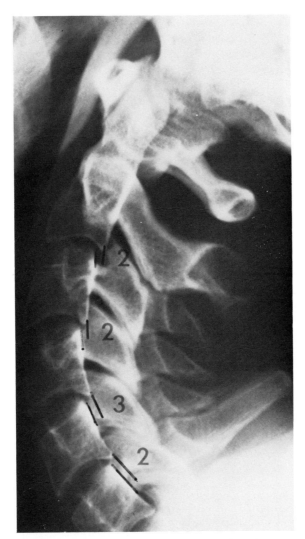

Figure 1.39. Extension lateral radiograph demonstrating the normal amount of "step-off" at each level. The *short solid lines* represent the posterior cortex of one vertebral body and the caudad extension of the posterior cortex of the next adjacent vertebra above. The number at each level is the actual amount of physiologic posterior "step-off" expressed in millimeters.

foramina and their margins. The transverse processes, being superimposed upon the pedicles, may normally, depending upon anatomic variations or minor deviations from the true oblique position, be projected into the intervertebral foramina, simulating a fracture fragment (Fig. 1.40). Normally, the articular mass of the vertebra above is superior and posterior with respect to the subjacent articular mass. Because the laminae are direct extensions of the articular masses (Fig. 1.27), the lamina of each vertebra is situated above and behind the

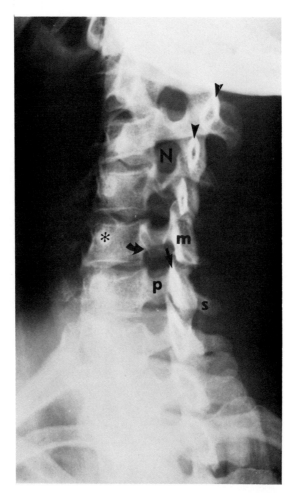

Figure 1.40. Oblique radiograph of the cervical spine in which the articular masses (*m*) are clearly delineated. At some levels, the laminae project through the articular masses as elongated densities that have a lucent center and are tapered at each end (*arrowheads*) and at other levels as tapered solid densities (*arrow*). This difference in appearance of the laminae is a normal variant. The transverse processes (*curved arrow*) are superimposed upon the pedicles (*p*). The spinous processes (*s*) are barely visible posteriorly and the pedicles of the opposite side project through the vertebral bodies as solid, round densities (*). The intervertebral (neural) foramina (*N*) are formed by adjacent portions of contiguous vertebrae.

subjacent lamina. In the oblique projection, laminae are normally seen "end-on" or in cross-section and they appear as oval-shaped densities with tapered superior and inferior ends seen through the density of the articular mass (Figs. 1.40 and 1.41). The lateral margin of a lamina represents its external cortex and the medial margin represents its internal cortex. Normally, the relationship of the laminae to each other is likened to that of "shingles on a roof," with the lamina above "covering" the subjacent lamina. If extended inferiorly, the long axis

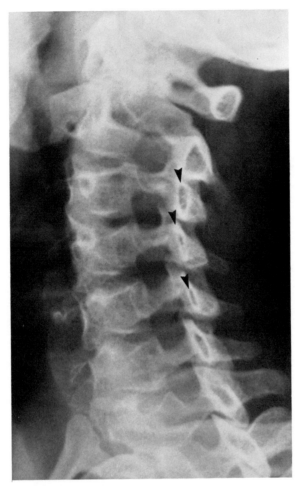

Figure 1.41. In an oblique projection that is steeper than Figure 1.40 (greater than 45°), the articular masses are not as clearly defined, but the laminae (*arrowheads*) which are clearly visible through the articular masses, reflect the normal position of the articular masses.

of a superior lamina should normally pass posterior to the external cortex of the subjacent lamina (Fig. 1.42). This fundamental anatomic concept remains valid even in improperly positioned oblique views where only the internal cortex of the laminae are radiographically visible (Fig. 1.43). The "shingles on a roof" concept is invaluable in the evaluation of oblique views obtained with the patient supine and which are characterized by image distortion due to the short target-film distance and the rather steep tube angulation required to obtain this view (Fig. 1.44). In oblique projections in which the relationship of the articular masses and interfacetal joints are clearly seen (Fig. 1.45), the "shingling" alignment of the laminae is a relatively unimportant observation because the articular masses themselves are well demonstrated.

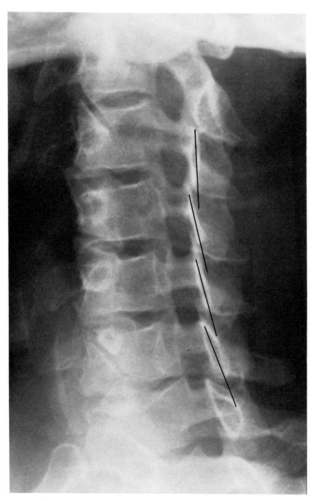

Figure 1.42. The *solid lines* represent the long axis of each lamina. When extended inferiorly, the long axis of the lamina projects above and behind the long axis of the subjacent lamina, thereby "covering" the subjacent lamina in the fashion of shingles on a roof. This normal alignment of the laminae reflects the normal alignment and relationship of the articular masses.

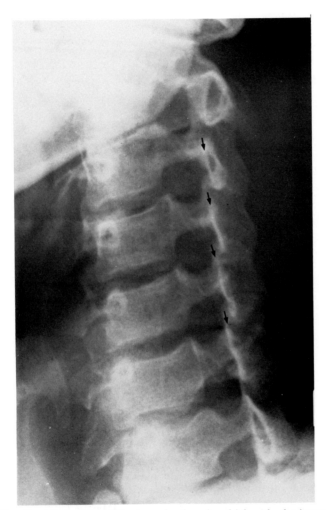

Figure 1.43.   In this shallow oblique projection, in which only the internal (medial) laminar cortex (*arrows*) is visible, the normal "shingle" relationship of the laminae (and, by inference, the articular masses) is established.

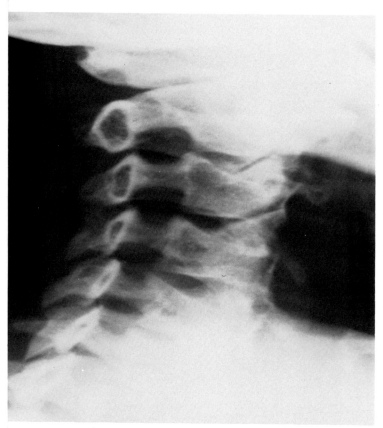

Figure 1.44. Oblique radiograph of the cervical spine obtained with the patient supine. In spite of the distortion and magnification, the normal "shingle" alignment of the laminae is clearly established.

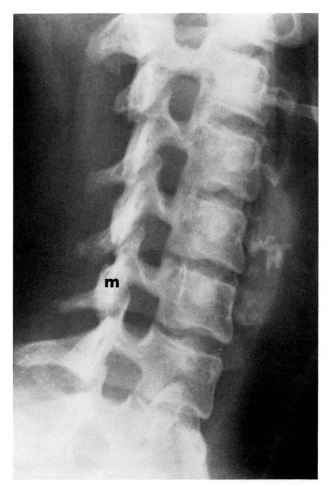

Figure 1.45. Oblique radiograph of the cervical spine in which the articular masses (*m*) are clearly seen to be normally aligned. In this instance, the inability to delineate the laminae is of no consequence.

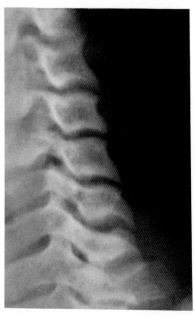

Figure 1.46.   Normal pillar (Weir) view of the left articular masses.

The oblique radiograph of the cervical spine is extremely useful regardless of patient positioning, and there is little justification to obtain a repeat oblique projection for positional reasons alone.

The pillar (15) view (Fig. 1.46) is designed to demonstrate the individual lateral masses in the coronal plane. This projection is particularly important in the detection of acute fractures of the lateral mass, i.e., the "pillar" fracture. The pillar view is made with the patient supine and the head in maximum rotation in the direction opposite the side to be examined in order to eliminate superimposition of the mandible and face upon the lateral masses. The x-ray tube is angled 35° caudad with the central beam centered 2 cm from the midline to the injured side. The central beam is centered at the level of the thyroid cartilage. If possible, depending upon the condition of the patient, the lateral masses of the opposite side should be examined by simply reversing the rotation of the head and the tube centering. An alternative method of obtaining a satisfactory pillar view has been suggested by Edeiken (19) when the patient is unable to rotate the head. Under these conditions, the examination is made with the patient erect, if possible, and with the central beam directed posteroanterior, angled cephalad approximately 35°, and centered just above the seventh spinous process.

Chapter 2

Radiographic Examination[a]

GENERAL CONSIDERATIONS

The extent of the radiographic examination of the cervical spine depends upon the patient's clinical condition, including neurologic status and, to a lesser degree, the type and magnitude of the causative force.

The plain-film study is the basic examination of the patient with acute cervical spine trauma. The radiographic dictum "one view is no view" is nowhere more apt than in the roentgenographic evaluation of acute cervical spine injury. A minimum of two views, preferably obtained in perpendicular planes, is essential. This principle applies particularly to the unconscious or polytraumatized patient in whom the entire radiographic study of the cervical spine must be obtained with the patient supine. Thus, it is a fact that the condition of the patient dictates the type of radiographic examination.

In every instance, the examination must cover the area from the base of the skull through the seventh cervical segment. Every reasonable attempt, consistent with the patient's condition, must be made to visualize the lower cervical segments in the initial plain-film study. If the seventh cervical vertebra is not adequately visualized, the cervical spine cannot be "cleared" until the lower cervical segments are completely visualized by either plain-film tomography or computed tomography.

The importance of the quality of the radiographic study cannot be overemphasized. The study must not only be of optimum technical quality in order to demonstrate both soft tissue and bone, but it must also be free of motion artifacts which can obscure subtle radiographic signs of injury. Because the superimposed density of the shoulders may obscure the cervicothoracic junction, it is frequently necessary to

---

[a]This chapter is taken largely from Harris, J.H., Jr.: Radiographic evaulation of spinal trauma. *Orthop. Clin. North Am.* 17:75–86, 1986. Reprinted with permission from W.B. Saunders Co.

use special radiographic projections and techniques to ensure adequate visualization of this area.

Patients requiring radiographic examination of the cervical spine may be described in two general groups: those who are less severely injured and those who are severely injured. The less severely injured patient with acute cervical spine trauma is usually characterized as being alert, conscious, able to cooperate, may be ambulatory, and has nonspecific signs and symptoms relative to the cervical spine that may or may not coexist with other relatively minor injuries. These patients should have the basic (standard, "routine") radiographic examination of the cervical spine.

The severely injured patient is usually characterized as being one who is unconscious, has obvious clinical signs of cervicocranial trauma, has a myelopathy, may be paralyzed, or is polytraumatized. The clinical condition of this group of patients usually requires that the basic radiographic examination of the cervical spine be modified to a "limited" study consisting of anteroposterior and supine lateral projections. Obviously, the distinction of these two groups of patients with acute cervical spine injury is a matter of individual clinical judgment. The importance of this clinical distinction is that the radiographic study must be modified to accommodate the condition of the patient yet be sufficiently comprehensive to be radiographically diagnostic.

The initial plain-film examination must be evaluated by a radiologist or other appropriately qualified physician prior to obtaining additional projections or using other imaging techniques.

THE BASIC (STANDARD, "ROUTINE") EXAMINATION

The basic radiographic examination of the cervical spine is indicated for patients with clinically less severe acute injuries of the cervical spine. This study should include the anteroposterior, "open-mouth," lateral, and oblique projections. As previously stated, the lateral radiograph must cover the base of the skull through C_7, and every reasonable attempt, consistent with the patient's condition, must be made to visualize all seven cervical segments (Fig. 2.1).

Oblique projections are included in the basic study in order to visualize the intervertebral foramina and their bony margins, to show the uncinate processes of the vertebral bodies differently than as seen in the anteroposterior projection, and to evaluate the integrity and orientation of the articular masses and their laminae. The most significant radiographic observation to be made in the oblique projection is the normal "shingling" orientation of the laminae (Fig. 1.42) or of the articular masses.

The basic examination must be reviewed by a radiologist or other qualified physician before additional plain films are obtained or other imaging techniques are employed. This is particularly true with respect to lateral flexion and extension views, which should be reserved only for those patients in whom there is historic or clinical evidence of a flexion or combined flexion-extension ("whiplash") injury, or radiographic signs suggesting anterior subluxation (hyperflexion sprain) (20,21).

The less severely injured patients are best examined in the radiology department with generally accepted, standard views and techniques. If possible, the patient should be examined at a target-film distance of 6 feet to eliminate magnification distortion. Depending on the patient's condition, examinations obtained at this distance may be made with the patient either standing or sitting. If the patient's condition precludes erect examination, perfectly diagnostic studies may

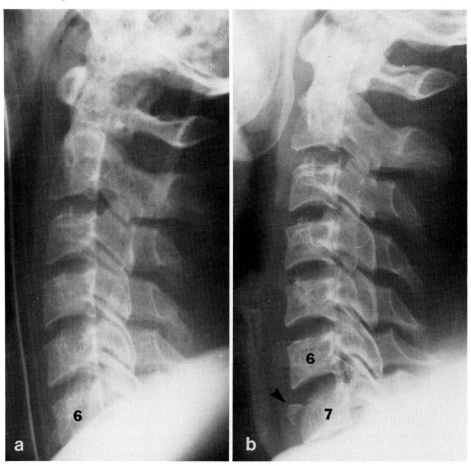

Figure 2.1. Lateral radiographs of the cervical spine illustrating the importance of visualization of all seven cervical segments in acute cervical spine injury. The density of the shoulders on the initial lateral radiograph (*a*) obscures the acute wedge fracture of C₇ (*arrowhead*) that is demonstrated on the lateral examination in which all seven cervical vertebral bodies are visible (*b*).

be obtained with the patient supine and at a target-film distance as short as 40 inches.

If, in the erect lateral radiograph, the lower cervical segments are obscured by the superimposed density of the shoulders, and assuming the patient has no contraindicating associated upper extremity injury, the shoulders can frequently be sufficiently distracted by the simple expediency of having the patient hold heavy weights in each hand, as in the examination for acromioclavicular joint separation. If the patient must be examined supine, gentle cervical traction applied simultaneously through the scalp and the upper extremities will frequently provide adequate visualization of the lower cervical segments. However, as has been previously emphasized, cervical traction for diagnostic radiographic purposes is specifically contraindicated in the presence of an existing, known cervical spine injury.

THE "LIMITED" RADIOGRAPHIC EXAMINATION

The "limited" radiographic examination of the cervical spine, which usually consists of anteroposterior and lateral supine projections, is dictated by the patient's condition and is used primarily as a screening procedure in those patients clinically identified as being "severely injured." While the "limited" examination is primarily intended for screening purposes, it is frequently diagnostic; in those instances, no additional initial radiographic studies are required or indicated. If, however, the "limited" study is equivocal, nondiagnostic, or inconsistent with the pertinent clinical findings, additional plain-film studies should be obtained at the time of the initial examination. Plain-film tomography or computed tomography should also be utilized when clinically appropriate. If the patient's condition will permit, an open-mouth view should be included in the "limited" study in order to visualize the atlantoaxial articulation in frontal projection. Frequently, however, either because of associated craniofacial injury, unconsciousness, or prior intubation, the "open-mouth" projection is not obtainable. Of the projections that constitute the "limited" study, the supine horizontal-beam lateral is the most important and should be obtained prior to the application of head and upper extremity traction in order to preclude distracting an existing skeletal or soft tissue injury (22) (Fig. 2.2).

The initial "limited" examination of the cervical spine of the severely injured patient is usually obtained in the trauma center with either portable or fixed-distance equipment. Under these circumstances, the likelihood of the shoulders obscuring the cervicothoracic junction is great, and special effort must be made to visualize this area. Supine oblique projections of each side of the cervical spine (Fig.

1.44), even though slightly distorted because of short target-film distance magnification, are more likely to be of diagnostic quality and provide more useful information than the "swimmer's" (Twining) projection. An additional important feature of the supine oblique projections is that they can be obtained without additional movement of the patient's head or neck. The supine oblique projections are obtained with the patient recumbent. The cassette is placed as far as possible posterior to the neck and as far under the shoulders and posterolateral aspect of the skull as possible. The x-ray tube is off-centered to the opposite side of the neck and angled approximately 45° toward the cassette with the central beam centered on the posteroinferior margin of the thyroid cartilage (Fig. 2.3). Supine oblique projections demonstrate the posterolateral aspect of the vertebral bodies, the pedicles, and the laminae projecting through the articular masses (Fig. 2.4). When studied in conjunction with the anteroposterior radiograph, the mentally integrated composite image of the lower cervical spine

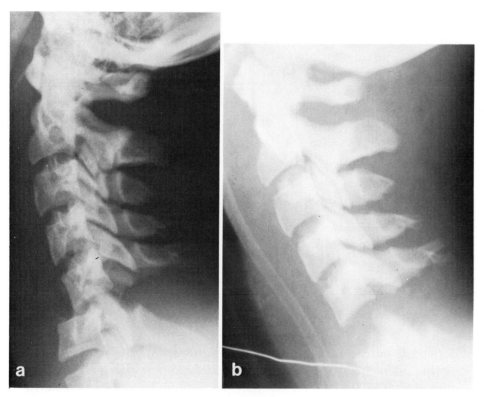

Figure 2.2. The effect of cervical traction on an unstable cervical spine injury. The initial supine lateral radiograph of the cervical spine (*a*) demonstrates an atypical bilateral interfacetal dislocation with obvious disruption of all of the soft tissues at the level of the injury. *b* shows the same patient after the application of only 10 pounds of cervical traction.

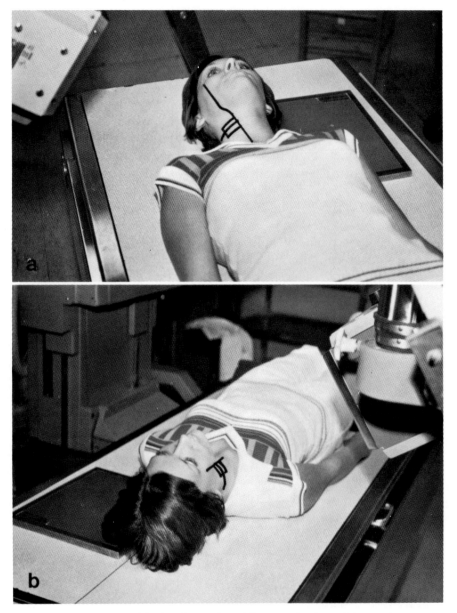

Figure 2.3.   Patient positioning for supine oblique projection of the cervical spine.

derived from the supine oblique and anteroposterior projections is usually adequate to establish or exclude major lower cervical spine injury. Should the supine oblique projections be nondiagnostic or equivocal, the cervical spine must remain immobilized until either plain-film tomography or computed tomography can be obtained.

The radiographic technique for the lateral projection must pro-

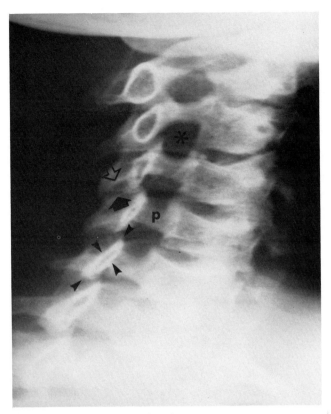

Figure 2.4.   Supine oblique radiograph. The posterolateral aspect of the vertebral bodies, the pedicles (*p*), the intervertebral foramina (*), and the interfacetal joints (superior facet, *open arrow; inferior facet, solid arrow*), and laminae (*arrowheads*) are clearly delineated.

vide maximum delineation of both the cervical vertebrae and the prevertebral soft tissues (Fig. 1.22). It is fundamentally important to delineate the prevertebral soft tissues because abnormal soft tissue swelling in the cervicocranium, which is visible only in the lateral projection, may be the most prominent radiographic sign of either a minimally displaced, subtle Jefferson bursting, dens, or "hangman's" (traumatic spondylolisthesis) fracture. Diffuse prevertebral soft tissue swelling throughout the cervical area and normally aligned cervical vertebrae in a patient with the acute central cord syndrome are the constant signs of hyperextension dislocation of the cervical spine and may be the only radiographic signs in 30% to 40% of patients with that injury (23,16).

Prior endotracheal or nasogastric intubation usually diminishes the value of the prevertebral soft tissues as an indicator of cervical spine injury. Deglutition (Fig. 2.5) or apnea, even in adults (Fig. 2.6), during the time of exposure of the horizontal-beam lateral radiograph may produce changes in the appearance of the cervical prevertebral soft tissues that mimic soft tissue swelling. If the patient is able to cooperate and has not been intubated, a horizontal-beam lateral radiograph obtained during vigorous inspiration provides optimum delineation of the prevertebral soft tissues.

Although the initial radiographic examination of severely injured patients is usually obtained in the trauma center with mobile equipment and less than optimum patient positioning, these conditions are neither an excuse for nor justification of radiographs that are *routinely* of inferior quality. It is precisely under the adverse conditions commonly attendant with the massively injured patient that radiographs of optimum quality must be the rule rather than the exception.

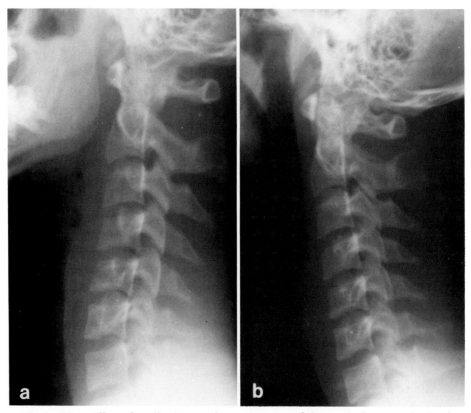

Figure 2.5. Effect of swallowing on the appearance of the cervical prevertebral soft tissues. The initial supine lateral radiograph (*a*) fortuitously coincided with patient swallowing. Note the absence of air in the naso-oropharynx and the presence of only two small collections of air in the distal hypopharynx. This study was interpreted as demonstrating diffuse prevertebral soft tissue swelling. An identical projection of the same patient (*b*) obtained 10 minutes later during inspiration demonstrates only normal cervical prevertebral soft tissues.

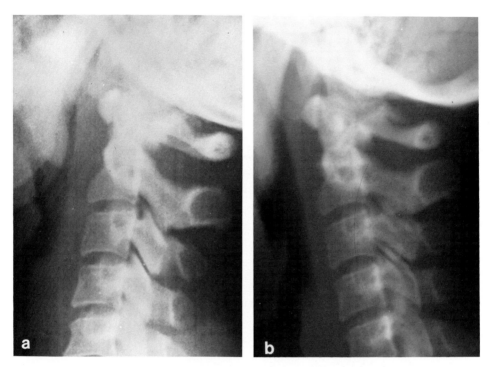

Figure 2.6.   Effect of hypoventilation (or apnea) on the cervical prevertebral soft tissues of an adult. In the initial supine lateral radiograph (*a*), the prevertebral soft tissues appear diffusely swollen, suggesting a massive prevertebral hematoma. However, close inspection demonstrates very little air in the oro-hypopharynx, relective of breath holding in expiration (apnea). A similar examination obtained on the same patient a short time later during deep inspiration (*b*) demonstrates normal prevertebral soft tissues.

ADDITIONAL PROJECTIONS

The "pillar" view is specifically designed to visualize the cervical articular masses *en face* (Fig. 2.7). Miller et al. (24) contend that the five-film cervical spine examination is inadequate and advocate that the pillar view be included in the routine evaluation of acute cervical spine injuries. However, it is generally agreed that the pillar view should be reserved for those patients either clinically or radiographically suspected of having articular mass fractures. The justification for the latter opinion is to limit the patient motion required to obtain the "pillar" view only to those patients in whom this projection is indicated. The pillar view requires rotating the patient's head in one direction, off-centering the x-ray tube approximately 2 cm in the opposite direction and angling the central beam approximately 35° caudad centered at the level of the superior margin of the thyroid cartilage. Caudal angulation places the central x-ray beam parallel to the plane of inclination of the interfacetal joints in the mid and lower cervical spine and

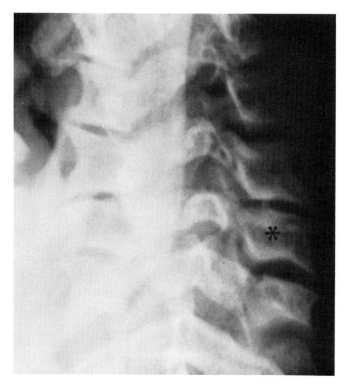

Figure 2.7.   Pillar view of normal left articular masses (∗).

the articular masses are thus projected *en face* because of the normal cervical lordosis. Rotation of the head is essential to eliminate superimposition of the mandible on the upper articular masses. Therefore, the patient must be able to rotate the head on command and the presence of a cervical spine injury must have been previously excluded on the basis of the original plain radiographs.

The "swimmer's" (Twining) view (Fig. 2.8) (25,26) is designed to visualize the cervicothoracic junction in patients in whom the density of the superimposed shoulders obscures the lower cervical segments in lateral projection. Optimum positioning for this projection requires that the patient be rotated slightly off the true lateral, with one upper extremity abducted 180° and extended cranially while the other upper extremity is extended posterocaudally. The amount of patient motion required to obtain the swimmer's view may be difficult, if not impossible, in the severely injured patient and is frankly contraindicated in patients in whom there is a high suspicion of injury to the cervicothoracic junction.

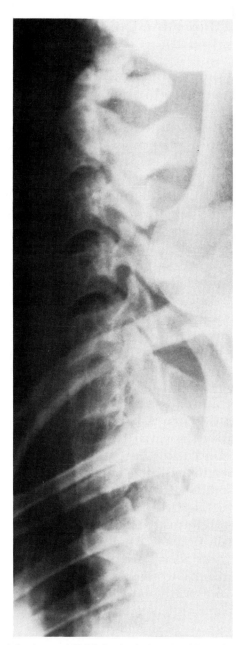

Figure 2.8.   Normal "swimmer's" (Twinning) view. In this optimal "swimmer's" projection, the lower cervical vertebral bodies are visualized, but the posterior elements are obscured by superimposed skeletal structures.

OTHER IMAGING TECHNIQUES
Tomography

Tomography of any form is not mandatory to assure a complete radiographic evaluation of *all* types of acute cervical spine injury. However, any facility intending to provide definitive management of acute cervical spine trauma *must have* tomographic capabilities available on a timely basis. Computed tomography (CT) is now considered essential for contemporary comprehensive assessment and management of acute spinal trauma (27–30).

Although some authors (29) advocate inclusion of thin-section plain-film tomography in the "routine" initial radiographic examination of acute cervical spine injuries, this is not a commonly accepted principle. Polydirectional tomography is superior to rectilinear tomography because its resolution provides sharper image definition. The disadvantages of polydirectional tomography include cost of the equipment, complexity and sophistication of operation, and limited clinical usefulness when compared with CT. For these reasons, polydirectional tomography is not widely available. Rectilinear tomography, on the other hand, is considerably less expensive, is frequently a component of a general diagnostic radiographic unit, and is simple to operate. Consequently, rectilinear tomography is more widely available. Although considered to be inferior to polydirectional tomography, rectilinear tomography is a reasonable alternative when polydirectional tomography is not available and when plain-film tomography is indicated for the evaluation of acute cervical spine trauma.

Plain-film tomography, either rectilinear or polydirectional, has the advantage of multisegmental spatial display in either the coronal (Fig. 2.9) or sagittal (Fig. 2.10) plane with sharper resolution than the sagittal and coronal reformatted CT images. Because plain-film tomography is traditionally oriented parallel to the longitudinal axis of the spine, it demonstrates axially oriented fractures (such as dens fractures) and the horizontally oriented avulsion fracture of the anterior arch of the atlas more clearly and reliably than computed tomography. Should the axial plane of the CT "slice" coincide with the plane of an axially oriented fracture, or should contiguous CT "slices" be parallel to but above and below such a fracture, the fracture defect would not be recorded. Secondary advantages of plain-film tomography are its availability and low cost. Disadvantages of plain-film tomography include the inability to provide axial images and the patient movement required to obtain images in any plane other than the coronal.

Computed tomography is the *tomographic* technique of choice (31,32) for evaluation of acute cervical spine trauma because of its fundamental axial display and because images in sagittal, coronal, or

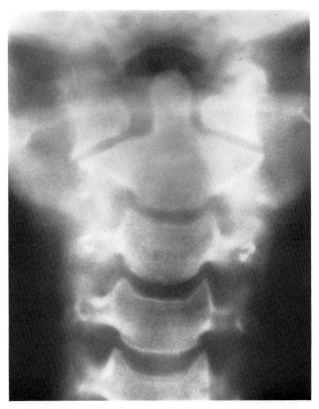

Figure 2.9. Normal polydirectional tomogram of the upper cervical segments in coronal projection demonstrating multisegmental dislplay and sharp definition of those structures at the level of the tomogram.

oblique planes can be reformatted without additional patient motion or additional radiation exposure. Patient radiation doses with CT are less than with plain-film tomography. The disadvantages of CT are cost, relatively limited availability, relatively poor resolution of the reformatted images, and possible failure to record axially oriented fractures. The advantages of CT far outweigh its disadvantages, however, and plain-film radiography combined with CT, when indicated, is the current standard of examination for evaluation of acute cervical spine injury.

Although tomography is not indicated for every type of acute cervical spine injury, it is reasonably indicated in any injury resulting in neurologic deficit, in fracture of the posterior arch of the cervical canal, and in every fracture with retropulsion of the posterior fragments. Within these general guidelines, Table 2.1 lists the specific types of cervical injuries for which tomography (plain-film or computed) can be expected to provide new or additional data, (i.e., the extent of bony injury, position of fragments, integrity of the spinal

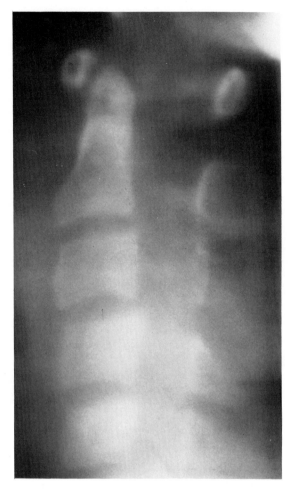

Figure 2.10. Normal polydirectional tomogram of the upper cervical segments in sagittal projection demonstrating multisegmental display and sharp definition of those structures at the level of the tomogram.

canal) relative to plain-film studies. Table 2.2 lists those injuries for which tomography should *not* be expected to provide new or additional data beyond that available from the plain-film studies.

It is essential that the reader not misconstrue Tables 2.1 and 2.2 to be lists of injuries for which tomography is "indicated" or "con-

Table 2.1.
Spinal Injuries for Which Tomography Is Useful

Flexion teardrop fracture
Pillar fracture
Jefferson bursting fracture, atlas
Burst fracture, lower cervical spine
Laminar fracture
Hyperextension fracture-dislocation

Table 2.2.
Cervical Spine Injuries for Which Tomography Is Usually Not Useful

Anterior subluxation (hyperflexion sprain)
Bilateral interfacetal dislocation
Simple wedge (compression) fracture
Clay shoveler's fracture
Unilateral interfacetal dislocation
Hyperextension dislocation
Extension teardrop fracture
Avulsion fracture of the anterior arch of the atlas
Posterior arch of atlas (isolated fracture)
Traumatic spondylolisthesis
Dens fractures

traindicated." The tables are not intended to be that rigid, but rather to serve as general guidelines for the efficient and effective use of time, money and absorbed radiation in the evaluation of acute cervical spine trauma. As stated, although tomography, particularly computed tomography with sagittal and coronal reformation may conceivably be useful in any acute cervical spinal injury, the relative clinical application of tomography can be reasonably assessed from the tables. Finally, tomography is specifically indicated when the plain-film study is equivocal or inconsistent with the patient's clinical signs and symptoms.

Three-Dimensional Computed Tomography (3-D CT)

With specially designed software, axial CT data obtained with zero gantry tilt can be converted into images which appear in three-dimensional format (Fig. 2.11). Available 3-D programs allow rotation of the images about any axis and permit transection of the image along the axial, coronal, or sagittal plane. In the latter two reformations, the observer sees the posterior arch as though from within the spinal canal. The conventional impression of 3-D CT is that it is simply a more easily comprehensible method of displaying complex anatomy or of demonstrating complex injuries to those less accustomed to the mental integration of multiplanar images.

Recent, preliminary application of 3-D CT to the evaluation of complex acute cervical spine injuries (33) has proven that 3-D CT does demonstrate clinically significant cervical spine injuries not otherwise appreciated by any other imaging modality, including high-resolution multiplanar CT. On the basis of this limited experience, 3-D CT has the potential of replacing sagittal and coronal reformation in the evaluation of acute cervical spine trauma. 3-D CT is specifically indicated in patients with complex injuries of the posterior arch and in any patient with cervical skeletal injury in whom the information derived from plain-film and multiplanar CT images is inconsistent with the patient's clinical findings.

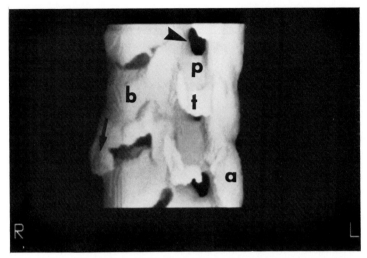

Figure 2.11. Three-dimensional CT of the midcervical spine demonstrating an osteo-phyte (*arrow*) that, on both plain films and CT, was interpreted as a fracture fragment. This image is slightly off-lateral and illustrates vertebral bodies (*b*), pedicles (*p*), trans-verse processes (*t*), intervertebral foramina (*arrowhead*), and articular masses (*a*).

Myelography

The indications for post-traumatic CT myelography are as varied and controversial as is the role of metrizamide CT myelography as a guide to patient management. The CT myelogram is infrequently utilized in the initial evaluation of acute cervical spine trauma (22,34–38).

Intrathecal administration of water-soluble contrast medium, combined with CT, provides direct visualization of the spinal cord, the cauda equina, and the nerve roots. It distinguishes between intra-medullary and extramedullary cord or root injury and obstruction to cerebral spinal fluid flow, and it demonstrates root avulsion, dural tear, or post-traumatic syringomyelia.

Small amounts (4 to 6 ml) of 170% water-soluble contrast medium are commonly employed. This may be introduced in the traditional myelographic technique, although patient motion required to do so usually precludes this approach. When clinical circumstances permit, the contrast material may be introduced into the lumbar subarachnoid space with the patient prone with or without fluoroscopic guidance. When CT myelography is indicated in cervical or upper thoracic inju-ries or the patient cannot be placed in the lateral decubitus or prone position, the contrast material may be introduced through a lateral C_1–C_2 approach with the patient supine. This technique is also useful for performing CT myelography following the application of cervical traction or immobilization. Actual scanning should be delayed for approximately 4 hours to permit reduction of the density of the metrizamide by redistribution and resorption (34–36,39).

Ultrasound

Sonography has no demonstrable application in the initial diagnosis of acute injuries of the spinal column, but has been reported useful in the intraoperative monitoring of the reduction of burst fractures of the thoracolumbar spine (40). Intraoperative sonography requires

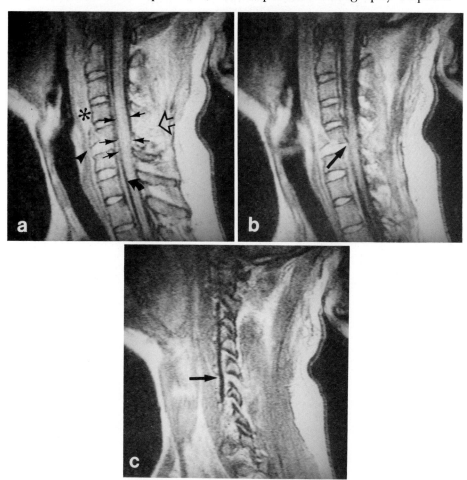

Figure 2.12. MR images of a flexion teardrop fracture of C_5 obtained on a Technicare 0.5 T system. The typical fracture fragment is clearly evident (*arrowhead*). Diffuse swelling of the spinal cord posterior to C_5 (*arrows*) is evident without the necessity of using intrathecal contrast. Diffuse prevertebral soft tissue swelling (*) and disruption of the posterior ligament complex between C_4 and C_5 (*open arrow*) are indicated by the high intensity signal. Hemorrhage, or edema, displaces the posterior longitudinal ligament (*curved arrow*) distal to the fracture.

Impaction of the posteroinferior corner of C_5 upon the ventral surface of the cord (*arrow*) is well demonstrated on the sagittal image obtained at a different level (*b*). An even more lateral image demonstrates the intact vertebral artery (*arrow*).

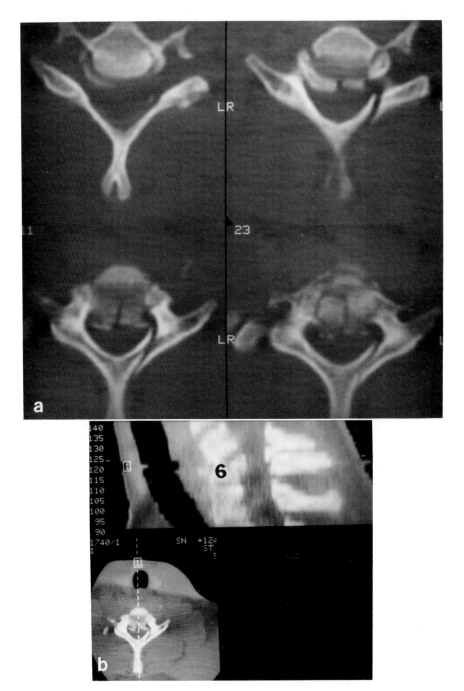

Figure 2.13. Axial (*a*) and sagittal reformatted (*b*) CT images of a "bursting" fracture of C_6. Cord compression by the retropulsed posterior central fragments (*arrow*) is clearly seen. On the sagittal SE 20/2000 pulse sequence (*c*) obtained on a GE 1.5 T Signa System, impingement of the retropulsed fragments (*arrowhead*), cephalad swelling of the cord, posterior separation of the posterior longitudinal ligament caudally, and localized prevertebral soft tissue swelling are clearly evident. In the T_2-weighted (SE 80/2000) image (*d*), the high-intensity signal within the cord (*arrowhead*) indicates the area of actual cord hemorrhage. The intact vertebral artery (*arrow*) is demonstrated in the lateral sagittal image (*e*) as is subluxation at the C_5–C_6 interfacetal joint (*open arrow*), the high-intensity signal of soft tissue edema (∗) and a tiny fracture of the superior facet of C_6 (*curved arrow*).

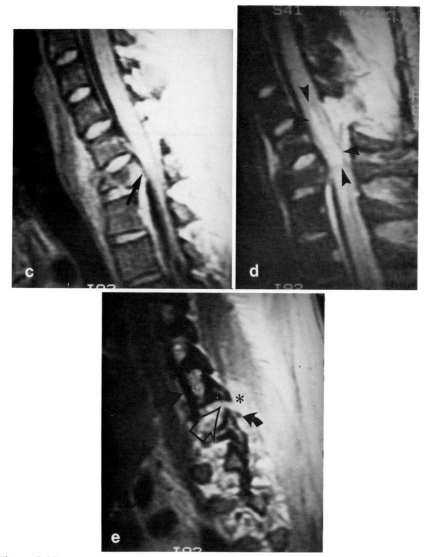

Figure 2.13. *c–e.*

laminectomy but provides real-time monitoring of the position of spinal fragments during and following reduction as well as the detection of such associated abnormalities as spinal cord hematoma.

Magnetic Resonance Imaging

As indicated earlier, and contrary to initial impressions, preliminary indications are that high-field strength MR will play a major role in the initial evaluation of acute cervical spine injuries. Further, it now seems reasonable that MR will become the single imaging technique which provides the most comprehensive information of acute spinal trauma (Fig. 2.12).

Earlier limitations to the use of MR in acute spinal trauma, particularly the cervical spine, included the lack of MR-compatible life-support or monitoring systems and the supposed inability of MR to record bone. Recently, life-support and patient monitoring systems that are MR-compatible have been developed, as have systems to maintain traction during MR examinations of the cervical spine.

High-field strength MR provides directly obtained images of the individual vertebrae and of the spinal column with greater resolution and definition than high-resolution CT sagittal or coronal reformations (Fig. 2.13). Because the spinal cord, as well as its surrounding structures, can be visualized directly by MR, it is reasonable to predict that MR imaging will replace metrizamide-CT in the evaluation of cord compression and obstructing intraspinal traumatic lesions.

Sequential MR imaging provides a qualitative assessment of cord injury not previously available by any other diagnostic technique.

Edema and/or hemorrhage of paraspinal soft tissues is clearly visualized by MR. At the appropriate sagittal levels, the vertebral arteries are clearly demonstrated by MR without the need for contrast injection. This is particularly valuable information, especially in those fractures and/or dislocations that may involve the foramen transvarsarium or the course of the vertebral arteries themselves.

At this time, MR is neither necessary nor indicated in the evaluation of those cervical spine injuries listed in Table 2.1 and probably should be reserved for those acute cervical spine injuries characterized by spinal canal involvement or that have produced a clinical neurologic deficit.

The principal disadvantages of MR are that small cortical fragments will not be recorded, the lack of its availability, and the relative unavailability of MR-compatible support and monitoring systems.

Chapter 3

A Practical Classification of Acute Cervical Spine Injuries[a]

Medical literature is replete with classifications of acute cervical spine injuries. The fact that so many classifications have been proposed and that none has gained general acceptance is indicative of their inability to satisfy the requirements of those working in this field.

The classification that follows is offered in the hope that it will provide a conceptual basis for understanding acute cervical spine injuries and facilitate an organized approach to the subject. In the hope that this classification will be meaningful and useful, it has a wider purpose than simply a listing of cervical spine injuries. It is applicable to the overwhelming majority of acute cervical spine injuries. It is simple, pragmatic, understandable and has equal application for the clinician and the theorist. The classification is based on terms and concepts commonly accepted by those working in the field and avoids the use of terms that are ambiguous, contradictory, or mutually exclusive.

Regarding acute cervical spine injuries, it is appropriate and useful that the mechanism of injury be the "common property or character" basis for segregation of these injuries into classes (groups or families). This notion is not new, having been the basis for many other attempts at classification of acute cervical spine injuries (15,21,41–52).

Biomechanical studies (18,50,51,53,54) and autopsy or cadaver experiments (43,55,56) have established the fundamental relationship between mechanism of injury—vector force—and acute injuries of the cervical spine. "The mechanism of injury is of major importance in the complete understanding of spine trauma" (18). In controlled laboratory experiments, "pure" vector forces—such as flexion, exten-

[a]This chapter is taken largely from Harris, J.H., Jr., Edeiken-Monroe, B., and Kopaniky, D.R.: A practical classification of acute cervical spine injuries. *Orthop Clin North Am* 17:15–30, 1986. Reprinted with permission from W.B. Saunders Co.

sion, vertical compression (axial load), lateral flexion, or a combination of these forces (simultaneous flexion and rotation or simultaneous extension and rotation) have been shown to produce injuries peculiar to each vector force or combination of forces. Pure or predominant vector forces may be further modified by simultaneous lateral flexion or shear forces, which helps to explain variations of the radiographic appearance of typical acute cervical spine injuries.

Clinically, the causative (vector) force of acute cervical spine injuries can only be inferred on the basis of historic, clinical, and radiologic evidence since the conditions of the mechanism of injury are certainly not controlled and usually not even directly observed. In all probability, the injury is a result of multiple simultaneous forces with one vector predominant rather than a single, pure force. The knowledge regarding the mechanisms of cervical spine injury obtained from controlled laboratory models may be reasonably applied to the injuries seen clinically because of the close pathologic and radiographic similarity of the experimental and clinical lesions. Therefore, it is reasonable to assume that acute cervical spine injuries are the result of either predominant or pure vector forces similar to those demonstrated in experimental models. If this assumption is valid, it seems reasonable to classify acute cervical spine injuries into groups of injuries caused by predominant or pure vector forces—that is, flexion, extension, vertical compression, or a combination thereof (simultaneous flexion and rotation or extension and rotation).

The radiographic appearance of acute cervical spine injury infrequently suggests a vertical distraction (the opposite of vertical compression) force. However, vertical distraction does not produce characteristic injuries, and the effects of this force are most often confined to the cervicocranium in the form of distractive atlanto-occipital disassociation and/or atlantoaxial disassociation.

The two-column concept of the spine (cervical) described by Holdsworth, (21,47) Louis (57), and White and Panjabi (18,58,59) (Fig. 3.1) is invaluable in understanding the pathophysiology of injuries occurring as a result of predominant flexion or extension vector forces. This concept defines the anterior column as comprising the "anterior elements," which include the anterior longitudinal ligament, vertebral body, intervertebral disk, and posterior longitudinal ligament. The posterior column consists of all the skeletal and ligamentous structures posterior to the posterior longitudinal ligament. Louis's (57) concept differs slightly in that he describes three pillars: "the anterior pillar formed by the vertebral body and the two pillars formed by the articular processes lying posteriorly." The anterior pillar and the intervertebral disk constitute the anterior column, and the paired posterior pillars, connected by the laminae and spinous process, form the pos-

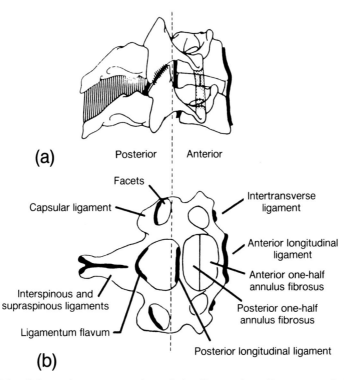

(a) Posterior | Anterior

Facets

Capsular ligament

Intertransverse ligament

Anterior longitudinal ligament

Anterior one-half annulus fibrosus

Interspinous and supraspinous ligaments

Posterior one-half annulus fibrosus

Ligamentum flavum

Posterior longitudinal ligament

(b)

Figure 3.1. Schematic representation of the "two column" concept of the spine. (From White, A. A., III, and Paujabi, M. M.: *Chemical Biomechanics of the Spine*. Philadelphia, J. B. Lippincott, 1978.)

terior column. More recently, Denis has redefined the spinal columns to include a middle column consisting of the "posterior wall of the vertebral body, the posterior longitudinal ligament and the posterior annulus fibrosus (60)." Although directed toward the thoracolumbar spine, the three-column concept may be relevant to certain lower cervical spine injuries. Its basic principle, however, reinforces the two-column concept, namely that during flexion through the sagittal plane (the Z axis), the anterior column is compressed and the posterior column is distracted (Fig. 3.2). Expressed differently, a predominant flexion vector force results in compression of the vertebral body and disk (anterior column) and simultaneous distraction of the posterior elements (posterior column).

Conversely, a hyperextension force causes simultaneous distraction of the anterior column and compression of the posterior column. The anterior and posterior columns, therefore, are affected reciprocally by both predominant flexion and extension forces. This fundamental concept obviates the need to attempt to classify acute cervical spine injuries by such terms as "compressive hyperflexion," "disruptive hyperflexion," "compressive hyperextension," "disruptive hyper-

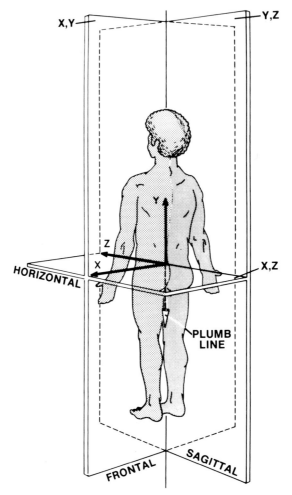

Figure 3.2.   Central coordinate system illustrating the planes of the X, Y, and Z axes. (From White, A.A., III, and Panjabi, M.M.: *Clinical Biomechanics of the Spine*. Philadelphia, J. B. Lippincott, 1978.)

extension," "compressive flexion," "distractive flexion," "flexion with or without compression," or "extension with or without compression" (42,52,61,62).

Only two additional facets remain to complete this concept of a method of classification of acute cervical spine injuries, both of which have general acceptance with respect to other skeletal injuries. The first is that different injuries may be caused by a single vector force. White and Panjabi expressed this concept by stating, "There are 'families' of injuries that result from identical or similar mechanisms of injury" (18). The second is that it is reasonable to assume a direct relationship between the magnitude of causative force and the type of injury, that is, the greater the force, the more severe the injury.

Finally, the literature, as well as clinical reality, provides commonly accepted terms for specific acute cervical spine injuries. A classification of such injuries requires only the assignment of this terminology to groups or families of injuries based on the recognized mechanism of injury.

The following classification (Table 3.1) is based on injuries, or families (groups) of injuries, generally accepted to be caused by predominant vector forces or combinations of such forces, as determined by the literature references cited after each group. Terms used to identify or describe each type of injury are those commonly employed clinically and experimentally.

Each predominant vector force is defined, both descriptively and with respect to the "central coordinate system" (see Fig. 3.2) (18,50,61). The generally accepted pathologic and radiologic descriptions of each specific type of acute cervical spine injury are provided, as is an illustration of the typical radiographic appearance of each injury.

Table 3.1.
Cervical Spine Injuries: Mechanism of Injury

Hyperflexion
    Anterior subluxation (hyperflexion sprain)
    Bilateral interfacetal dislocation
    Simple wedge (compression) fracture
    Clay shoveler's (coal shoveler's) fracture
    Flexion teardrop fracture

Simultaneous Hyperflexion and rotation
    Unilateral interfacetal dislocation (locked vertebra)

Simultaneous Hyperextension and rotation
    Pillar fracture

Vertical compression
    Jefferson bursting fracture
    Burst (bursting, dispersion, axial loading) fracture

Hyperextension
    Hyperextension dislocation (hyperextension sprain or strain)
    Avulsion fracture of the anterior arch of the atlas
    Extension teardrop fracture of the axis
    Fracture of posterior arch of atlas
    Laminar fracture
    Traumatic spondylolisthesis (hangman's fracture)
    Hyperextension fracture--dislocation

Lateral flexion
    Uncinate process fracture

Injuries caused by diverse or imprecisely understood mechanisms
    Atlanto-occipital disassociation (extension-flexion)
    Odontoid fractures

CLASSIFICATIONS OF INJURIES

Hyperflexion

Flexion (hyperflexion) injuries are caused by a pure, or predominant, forward rotation and/or translation of a cervical vertebra in the sagittal plane, that is, the Z axis (Fig. 3.2). Flexion injuries are the result of simultaneous compression of the anterior column and distraction of the posterior column of the spine. Injuries in this group may be pure soft tissue, pure skeletal, or a combination.

Anterior Subluxation (Hyperflexion Sprain). Anterior subluxation is characterized in the lateral projection by a hyperkyphotic angulation of the cervical spine localized to the level(s) of the ligamentous disruption (Fig. 3.3) (21,42,45,47,51,63–75). Anterior subluxation is, by definition, limited to disruption of the posterior ligament complex (21) and has a 30 to 50% incidence of "delayed instability" (63) consequent to failure of ligamentous healing.

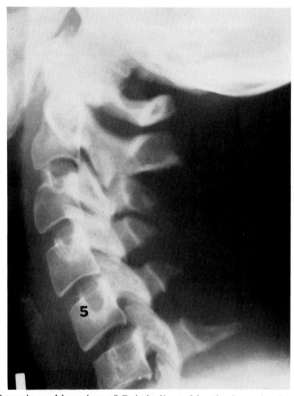

Figure 3.3.   Anterior subluxation of C_5 is indicated by the hyperkyphotic angulation at the C_5–C_6 level secondary to anterior rotation and translation of C_5, resulting in widening of the interspinous and interlaminar space, subluxation of the C_5–C_6 interfacetal joints, and posterior widening and anterior narrowing of the fifth intervertebral disk space.

Disruption of the posterior ligament complex is (*a*) the pathologic finding of anterior subluxation, (*b*) an integral part of all flexion injuries except the clay shoveler's fracture, and (*c*) an inherent component of unilateral interfacetal dislocation (43).

Bilateral Interfacetal Dislocation. Bilateral interfacetal dislocation is dislocation of each interfacetal (facetal, facet, apophyseal) joint at the same level and can occur anywhere in the lower cervical spine from C_2 through C_7 (42,43,48,51,61,66,76–79). With hyperflexion, all of the ligamentous structures at the level of the injury are disrupted, allowing anterior displacement of the involved vertebra to the degree that the articular masses of the dislocated vertebra pass superiorly and anteriorly over the subjacent articular masses and come to rest in the inferior portion of the corresponding intervertebral foramina. Radiographically, bilateral interfacetal dislocation is characterized by anterior displacement of the dislocated segment a distance equal to at least one-half the anteroposterior diameter of a cervical vertebral body. The inferior facets of the dislocated vertebra lie anterior to the superior facets of the subjacent segment (Fig. 3.4).

Although impaction fractures of the margins of the dislocated facetal joint frequently occur during dislocation, the fragments are typically small and usually of no clinical significance.

Bilateral interfacetal dislocation is occasionally referred to as the "double locked" vertebra (42,52,62,80), thereby creating the impression of a stable (locked) injury. Pathologically, frank bilateral interfacetal dislocation is acutely unstable because of the skeletal (bilateral interfacetal dislocation) and soft tissue (complete ligamentous) disruption at the level of injury. For these reasons, double locked vertebra is not an apt synonym for bilateral interfacetal dislocation, and its use is to be avoided.

Simple Wedge (Compression) Fracture. Hyperflexion of sufficient force to cause impaction of one vertebra against the subjacent vertebra may cause a simple wedge fracture (42,48,51,81,82). This fracture is typically characterized radiographically by impaction of the superior end plate and impaction and angulation of the anterior cortical margin of the vertebral body. Consequently, vertical stature of the anterior aspect of the involved centrum is lost (Fig. 3.5). Pathologically, in addition to the vertebral body fracture, the posterior ligament complex is disrupted.

Clay Shoveler's (Coal Shoveler's) Fracture. The clay shoveler's fracture is an avulsion fracture of the spinous process of C_7, C_6, or T_1, in that order of prevalence (76,83). It occurs when the head and upper cervical segments are forced into flexion against the opposing action of the interspinous and superspinous ligaments. Radiographically, the clay shoveler's fracture is characterized by an oblique fracture limited to the spinous process of the involved vertebra (Fig. 3.6).

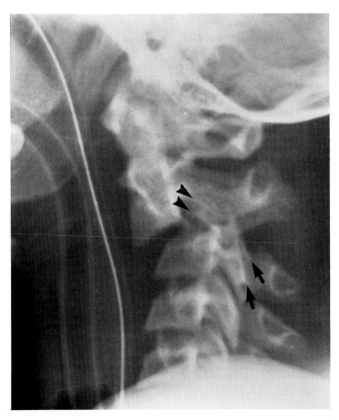

Figure 3.4.   Bilateral interfacetal dislocation of C_2. The axis is rotated and translated anteriorly to the degree that the body of C_2 is displaced anteriorly with respect to the body of C_3 at a distance greater than 50% of the anteroposterior diameter of the vertebral body. The inferior facets of the axis (*arrowheads*) are completely dislocated anteriorly with respect to the subjacent superior facets of C_3 (*arrows*).

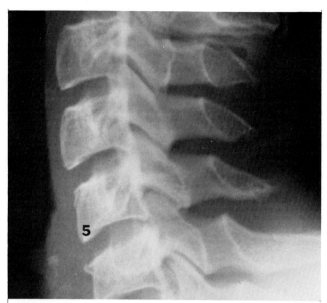

Figure 3.5. Simple wedge (compression) fracture of the bodies of C_5 and C_6 is characterized by decreased anterior vertical height and disruption (C_5) and buckling (C_6) of the anterior cortex of the centrum.

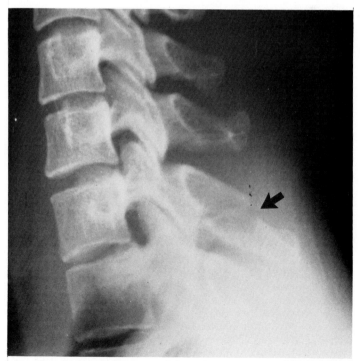

Figure 3.6. Clay shoveler's fracture of the spinous process of C_6 (*arrow*).

Flexion Teardrop Fracture.   Pathologically, the flexion teardrop fracture is characterized by complete disruption of all of the ligaments and the intervertebral disk at the level of injury, by disruption of the interfacetal joints, and by a large triangular fragment consisting of the anterior inferior aspect of the involved vertebral body (42,46,55,81,84,85).

The lateral cervical radiograph reflects the pathologic features of the flexion teardrop fracture. In addition, the cervical spine is usually in a flexed attitude above the level of the injury, and prevertebral soft tissue swelling is invariably present (Fig. 3.7).

Clinically, the flexion teardrop fracture is the most devastating of all flexion injuries, being associated, by definition, with the acute ante-

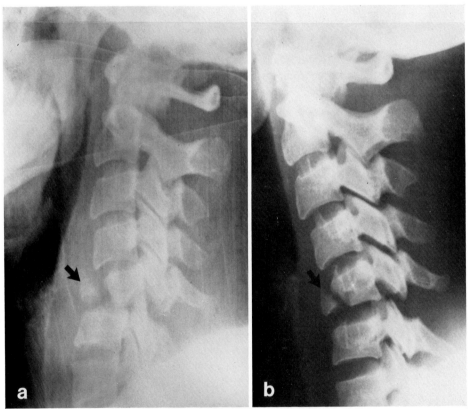

Figure 3.7.   Flexion teardrop fracture of C₅. In the initial lateral radiograph (*a*), the hyperkyphotic angle at the C₅–C₆ level, marked increase in interspinal and interlaminar spaces, dislocation of the interfacetal joints, and rotation of C₅ all reflect the causative flexion vector force. The intervertebral disk space is narrowed, reflecting disk disruption. The centrum is intact except for the single large triangular ("teardrop") fragment (*arrow*) in its anterior inferior corner. The lateral radiograph obtained after skeletal traction (*b*) confirms all the pathologic features of the flexion teardrop fracture (*arrow*) seen on the initial study and more clearly demonstrates the complete ligamentous disruption at the C₅–C₆ level.

rior cervical cord syndrome consisting of "immediate, complete paralysis with hypesthesia and hypalgesia to the level of the lesion together with the preservation of touch, motion, position, and vibration sense" (86).

Simultaneous Hyperflexion and Rotation

Unilateral Interfacetal Dislocation (Locked Vertebra).   Unilateral interfacetal dislocation is the result of simultaneous flexion and rotation vector forces (43,48,52,53,61,77,87–91). Pathologically, unilateral interfacetal dislocation consists of dislocation of a facetal joint at one level on the side opposite that of the direction of rotation. This dislocated articular mass is displaced anterior to the subjacent mass and becomes wedged in the inferior portion of the intervertebral foramen. The posterior ligament complex and the capsule of the dislocated facetal joint are disrupted. The anterior and posterior longitudinal ligaments and the disk are disrupted or attenuated.

Unilateral interfacetal dislocation may be associated with an impaction fracture of either of the articular masses of the dislocated interfacetal joint. The fracture fragment usually is small and, like the fractures typically associated with bilateral interfacetal dislocation, is not a major component of the injury.

Because of the position of the dislocated articular mass wedged in the intervertebral foramen between the subjacent vertebral body and ular mass during hyperextension and rotation (52,62,66,92–96). locked vertebra, which correctly implies a mechanically stable injury.

In the lateral radiograph, unilateral interfacetal dislocation is characterized by forward displacement of the dislocated vertebra a distance less then one-half of the anteroposterior diameter of a cervical vertebral body. In addition, the rotary component is evidenced by lack of superimposition of the paired articular masses at the level of dislocation and above. Because of the rotation, the articular masses on the side of dislocation are superimposed on the vertebral bodies (Fig. 3.8). In the anteroposterior projection, rotation is evidenced by the spinous processes being displaced from the midline toward the side of the dislocated interfacetal joint at the level of the dislocation and above.

Simultaneous Hyperextension and Rotation

Pillar Fracture.   The pillar fracture (compressive extension—CE stage 1 (61)) is a vertical fracture of the articular pillar (mass) resulting from impaction of the involved mass by the ipsilateral superior articular mass during hyperextension and rotation (52,62,66,92–96).

On the lateral radiograph (Fig. 3.9), the fracture is indicated by a lack of superimposition of the posterior margins of the articular masses at the level of injury secondary to retropulsion of the posterior fragment ("double outline" sign) (94) and, frequently, by a visible fracture line in the inferior facet of the involved mass. On anteroposterior projection (Fig. 3.9), the fracture may be evidenced by a fracture line in the lateral column. The pillar fracture is best demonstrated, however, in the oblique and pillar projections.

Vertical Compression. Vertical compression (axial loading) is a force delivered to the longitudinal (Y) axis (see Fig. 3.1) of the spinal column at the instant the cervical spine is straight, i.e., neither flexed nor extended (21,48,50–52,62). The force is usually transmitted to the spine through the occipital condyles from a blow to the top of the skull but may be transmitted through the pelvis.

Injuries attributable to vertical compression are the Jefferson bursting fracture of the atlas (97) and the burst, or bursting (43), fracture of the lower cervical spine.

Jefferson Bursting Fracture. As originally described (98), this fracture consists of bilateral fractures of both the anterior and posterior

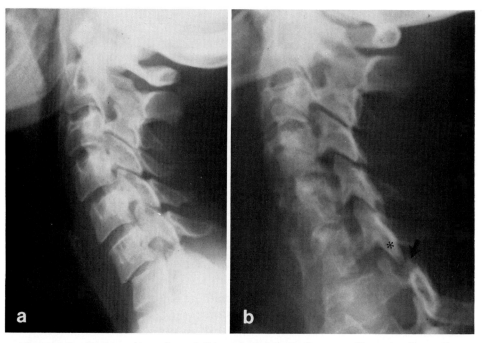

Figure 3.8. Unilateral interfacetal dislocation of C_6. In the neutral lateral radiograph (*a*), flexion is indicated by forward rotation and translation of C_6 a distance less than one-half the transverse diameter of a cervical vertebral body, by increased interspinous space, and by a dislocated interfacetal joint. The rotatory component is evidenced by the interfacetal joint dislocation and the ipsilateral forward displacement of articulating masses and their interfacetal joints from the level of the injury cephalad and by the clearly visible intervertebral foramina at the C_2–C_3 level. The left anterior oblique radiograph (*b*) demonstrates the dislocated facetal joint, with the inferior articulating process of C_6 (*) seated in the intervertebral foramen anterior to the fractured superior articulating process of C_7 (*arrow*).

arches of C_1. Computed tomography (CT) has shown that the Jefferson fracture may result from a single break in each ring. Radiographically, the Jefferson fracture is characterized, in frontal projection, by bilateral lateral displacement of the articular masses of C_1 (Fig. 3.10). In the lateral projection, the anterior arch fracture is rarely seen, whereas the posterior arch fracture is commonly demonstrated. The diagnosis of a Jefferson bursting fracture can be established on the anteroposterior projection of the atlantoaxial articulation alone. However, in lateral projection, the Jefferson fracture cannot be distinguished from the isolated hyperextension fracture of the posterior arch of the atlas. Cervicocranial prevertebral soft tissue swelling is a common secondary sign of a Jefferson fracture, but is not associated with the isolated fracture of the posterior arch of C_1.

Burst Fracture. The burst, or bursting, fracture of the lower cervical spine was originally described as a comminuted fracture of the vertebral body with variable retropulsion of the posterior body fragments into the spinal canal (vertical compression—VC stage 3) (61,66,81,98). Until the advent of CT, this fracture was believed to be confined to the centrum. CT has demonstrated that a posterior arch fracture, usually involving the lamina, is invariably present. Radiographically, the burst fracture of the lower cervical spine is characterized in lateral projection by comminution of the centrum with varying degrees of retropulsion of the posterior body fragments. Typically, the cervical spine is straight, and the alignment of the posterior elements

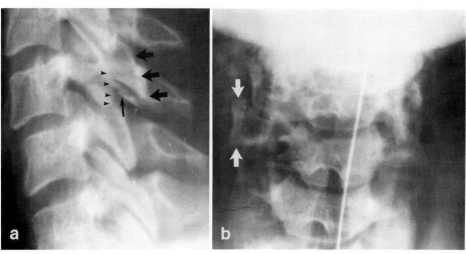

Figure 3.9. "Pillar" fracture, right articular mass, C_4. The lateral radiograph (*a*) shows the "double outline" sign resulting from the posterior location of the posterior cortical margin of the retropulsed fragment of the fractured articular mass (*arrows*) with respect to the contralateral posterior cortical margin (*arrowheads*) and the fractured inferior articulating facet (*vertical arrow*). In the anteroposterior projection (*b*), the lateral mass of C_4 is laterally displaced (*arrows*), disrupting the right lateral column.

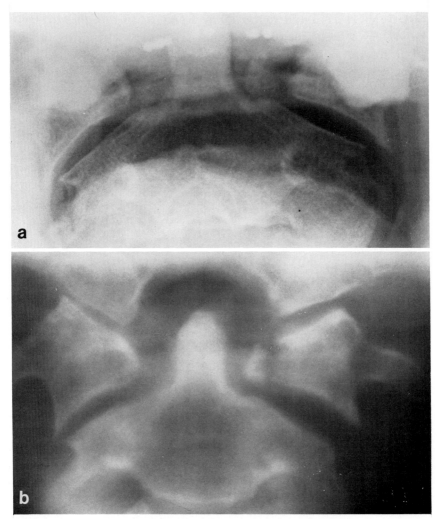

Figure 3.10. Bilateral lateral displacement of the articular masses of a Jefferson bursting fracture of the atlas seen in the "open-mouth" plain radiograph (*a*) and in a frontal tomogram (*b*). These projections also demonstrate an avulsion fracture of the left lateral mass of C$_1$ caused by the intact transverse atlantal ligament. The posterior arch fractures (*arrowheads*) are visible in the lateral radiograph (*c*). The axial computed tomogram of the atlas (*d*) demonstrates the single anterior arch fracture (*arrowhead*) and confirms bilateral lateral displacement of the articular masses, the avulsion fragments from the right lateral mass, and the bilateral posterior arch fractures (*curved arrows*).

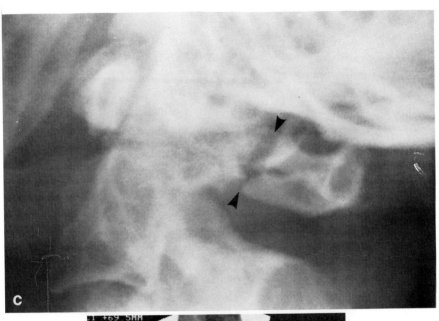

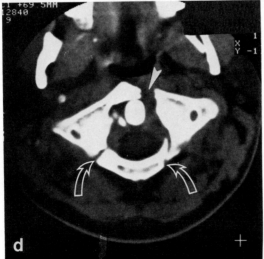

Figure 3.10. *c* and *d*.

is normal (Fig. 3.11*a*). A vertical fracture of the vertebral body is seen on the anteroposterior radiograph (Fig. 3.11*b*). The posterior arch fracture is only discernible on CT (Fig. 3.11*c*).

Some authors (18,51,99) consider the bursting fracture of the lower cervical spine and the flexion teardrop fracture described by Schneider and Kahn (85) to be variations of the same injury. The majority of authors, (41,43,47,48,50,52,66,81,100–103), however, make a distinction between the bursting fracture of the lower cervical spine and the flexion teardrop fracture on the basis of (*a*) the inferred mechanism of injury, (*b*) the neurologic findings, (*c*) the overall attitude of the cervical spine in general, and (*d*) the characteristics of the involved vertebra in particular on the lateral cervical radiograph.

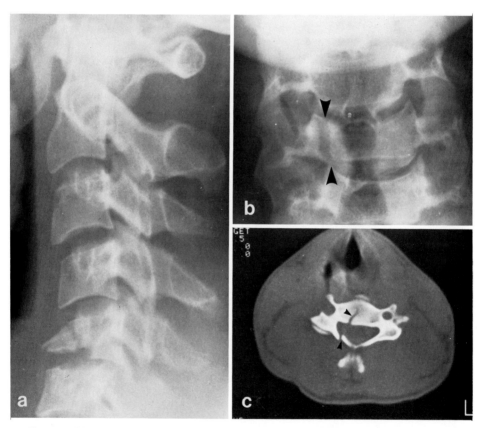

Figure 3.11. Burst (bursting, dispersion, vertical compression, axial loading) fracture of C$_5$ is characterized in lateral projection (*a*) by essentially straight orientation of the cervical vertebrae, comminution of C$_5$ centrum with retropulsion of its posterior fragments, and the absence of distraction of the posterior column. In the frontal projection (*b*), the burst fracture is characterized by a vertical fracture through the vertebral body (*arrowheads*). The axial CT (*c*) demonstrates the vertical body fracture and the invariably present posterior arch fracture (*arrowheads*).

Hyperextension

Extension (hyperextension) injuries are the opposite of flexion injuries. They result from a posterior rotation and/or translation of a cervical segment(s) in the sagittal plane (the Z axis). Depending on the direction and magnitude of the posteriorly directed vector force, any one of a family of cervical spine injuries, each with distinctive radiographic characteristics of a predominantly hyperextension mechanism, may result.

Hyperextension Dislocation (Hyperextension Sprain or Strain). Hyperextension dislocation (distractive extension—DE stage 2) (61) is a specific injury that has been produced experimentally in monkeys and in cadaver experiments; it has also been observed at autopsy (23,45,46,54,62,104–109).

Hyperextension dislocation has been described as the result of a direct posterior force impacting on the face and propelling the head and cervical spine into a hyperextension. Pathologically, the hyperextension force causes disruption of the anterior longitudinal ligament, posterior rotation and translation of the involved cervical segment, either horizontal disruption of the intervertebral disk or avulsion of the inferior end plate of the involved centrum from the superior margin of the disk, with a frequently associated fracture of the anterior aspect of the inferior end plate, and separation of the posterior longitudinal ligament from the subjacent vertebra. The posterior column assumes a kyphotic attitude as a result of anterior bulging of the ligamentum flavum and anterior angulation of the laminae. Consequently, the cervical cord is pinched both anteriorly and posteriorly, producing the characteristic acute central cervical cord syndrome. Following dissipation of the causative force, the spine returns to normal position and alignment.

Radiographically, hyperextension dislocation is uniformly characterized by the combination of normal alignment of the cervical vertebrae and diffuse prevertebral soft tissue swelling. A thin, horizontally oriented avulsion fracture arising from the anterior aspect of the inferior end plate of the involved vertebra may be present in approximately 60% of patients (Fig. 3.12). Vacuum defect and widened intervertebral disk space at the level of injury are other infrequent localizing signs (16).

Avulsion Fracture of the Anterior Arch of the Atlas. This rare injury (11,62,110) is a horizontal fracture of the anterior arch of the atlas caused by a hyperextension force against the intact longus colli muscles and the atlantoaxial ligament, both of which insert on, or inferior to, the anterior tubercle of the atlas. A horizontal fracture line of the anterior arch of C_1 and cervicocranial prevertebral soft tissue swelling are seen on the lateral radiograph (Fig. 3.13).

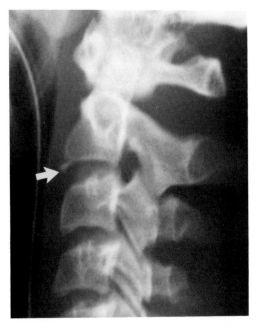

Figure 3.12.   Hyperextension dislocation of C$_2$ characterized by normal alignment of the cervical vertebrae and diffuse prevertebral soft tissue swelling. Avulsion of the ring apophysis of the axis (*arrow*) marks the dislocated segment.

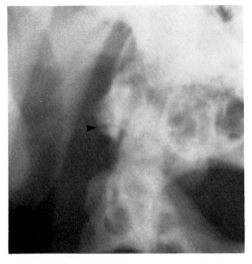

Figure 3.13.   Acute avulsion fracture of the anterior arch of the atlas (*arrowhead*).

Extension Teardrop Fracture of the Axis. The extension teardrop fracture (21,45,47,48,62,67) is a relatively large triangular fragment with its vertical height equal to or greater than its transverse width (Fig. 3.14). The separate fragment composes the anterior inferior corner of the body of the axis, which is avulsed by the intact anterior longitudinal ligament during hyperextension of the head and upper cervical spine. Extension teardrop fracture occurs most commonly in older patients with osteopenia or cervical spondylosis.

Fracture of the Posterior Arch of the Atlas. The isolated fracture of the posterior arch of the atlas (Fig. 3.15) is the result of compression of the posterior arch between the occiput and the heavy spinous process of the axis during hyperextension (62,66,98,99,112–115). This injury should be distinguished from the Jefferson bursting fracture by the absence of prevertebral soft tissue swelling in the cervicocranium, the absence of bilateral lateral displacement of the articular masses of C_1 on the "open-mouth" projection, and the absence of an anterior arch fracture.

Laminar Fracture. By definition, isolated laminar fractures (compressive extension—CE stages 1 and 2) (61) involve that portion of the posterior arch of the lower cervical vertebrae between the articular mass and the spinous process (62,116,117). This uncommon fracture

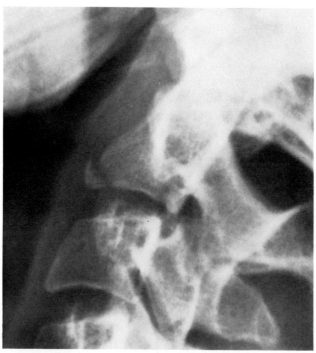

Figure 3.14. Hyperextension teardrop fracture of the axis. The vertical height of the characteristic separate fragment exceeds its horizontal width.

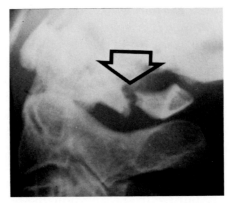

Figure 3.15.   Isolated fracture of the posterior arch of the atlas.

usually occurs in older patients with cervical spondylosis. Radiographically, laminar fractures are frequently subtle, are characterized by disruption of the laminae on lateral projection (Fig. 3.16), and are usually best identified by CT (Fig. 3.16).

   Traumatic Spondylolisthesis of the Axis (Hangman's Fracture). Traumatic spondylolisthesis in its usual and typical form is a bilateral fracture of the pars interarticularis of the axis (Fig. 3.17) caused by hyperextension force (2,18,47,62,66,81,99,112,118–120). Much less commonly, one or both fractures may involve the superior articulating facet and its subjacent bone or may be more anteriorly located at the junction of the posterior arch and posterior aspect of the axis centrum.

   Hyperextension Fracture-Dislocation.   Hyperextension dislocation (compressive extension—CE stages 4 and 5) (42,45,46,67,117,121) is a unique radiographic diagnostic problem because, even though caused by a predominantly hyperextension force, bilateral posterior arch disruption allows the circular hyperextension force to propel the

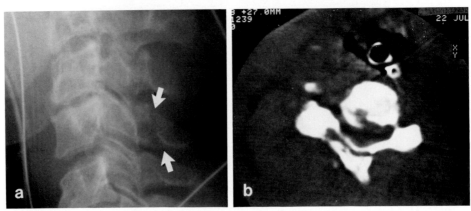

Figure 3.16.   Laminar fracture of C_4 in lateral projection (*a*) (*arrows*) and axial CT (*b*).

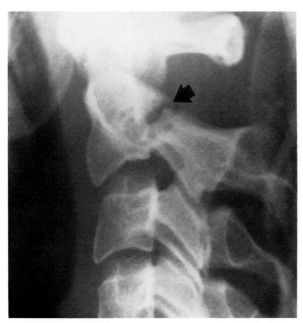

Figure 3.17. Traumatic spondylolisthesis of C_2 (hangman's fracture). The bilateral fractures (*arrow*) involve the pars interarticularis.

body of the involved vertebra anteriorly, thereby resembling a flexion injury on the lateral radiograph. Hyperextension fracture-dislocation is characterized by bilateral articular mass fractures or a mass fracture on one side and a contralateral facetal joint dislocation. Radiographically, in lateral projection, the anatomy of the posterior elements at the level of injury is completely disorganized because of the fracture and/or dislocation, and the centrum of the involved vertebra is slightly anteriorly displaced. In anteroposterior projection, the lateral columns are disrupted at the level of injury (Fig. 3.18). Oblique radiographs are invaluable in delineation of the posterior element pathology.

Lateral Flexion

Lateral flexion (bending) (18,42,50–52,61,62,122,123) is translation or tilt in the X axis (Fig. 3.2) and rarely occurs as a dominant injury vector force to the cervical spine. Lateral flexion is more commonly seen as modifying a primary vector force, such as is illustrated in Figure 3.19, where the marked lateral displacement of the left articular mass component of the Jefferson bursting fracture and the compression fractures of the left lateral aspect of the body of the axis are best explained as the result of simultaneous vertical compression and left lateral flexion of the head and cervicocranium.

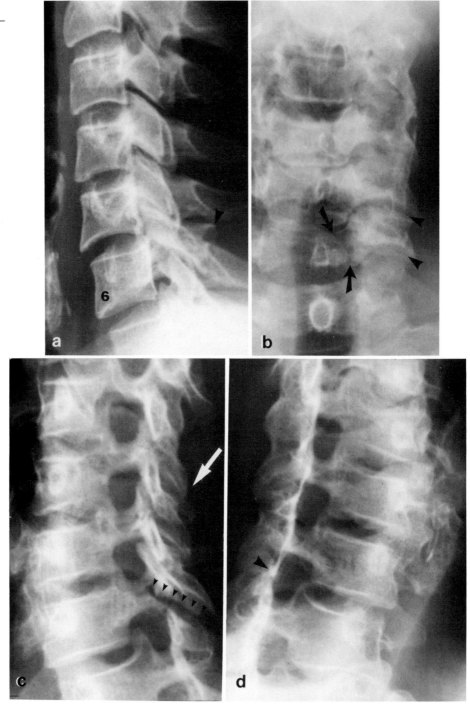

Figure 3.18. Hyperextension fracture dislocation of C_6. In lateral projection (*a*), the body of C_6 is anteriorly translated with respect to C_7. The C_6 articular masses and adjacent interfacetal joints are disorganized, resulting in the "absent facet" sign. A laminar fracture of C_6 (*arrowhead*) is also present. In the frontal projection (*b*), the left articular mass of C_6 is rotated so that the corresponding interfacetal joints are visible (*arrowheads*), as is a left laminar fracture (*arrows*). The fracture involving the left lamina, articular mass, and pedicle (*arrowheads*) is seen in the left anterior oblique projection (*c*), and the incompletely dislocated ("perched") C_6–C_7 interfacetal joint (*arrowhead*) is seen in the right anterior oblique projection (*d*). The left articular mass fracture and the contralateral (right) disrupted interfacetal joint permit anterior translation of the involved vertebra, resulting in the seemingly inappropriate anterior translation of the vertebral body in a hyperextension injury.

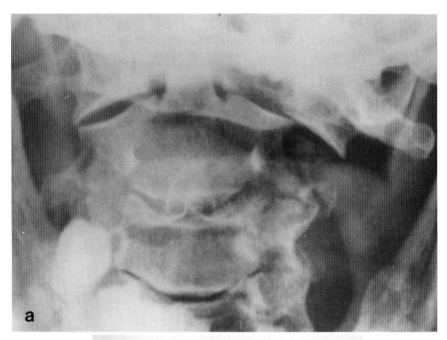

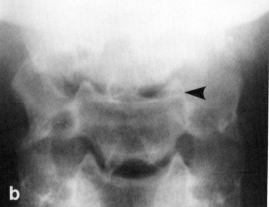

Figure 3.19. (*a*) A primary vector force resulted in eccentric lateral displacement of the left articular mass of the Jefferson bursting fracture and the comminuted fracture of the lateral mass of the axis and of C₃. (*b*) Acute transverse fracture of a left uncinate process (*arrowhead*) secondary to lateral tilt vector force.

Uncinate Process Fracture. Fracture of the uncinate process (Fig. 3.19) is the only discrete cervical spine fracture attributable to lateral flexion.

Injuries Caused By Diverse Or Imprecisely Understood Mechanisms

Atlanto-occipital Disassociation (Extension-Flexion). Atlanto-occipital disassociation (62,69,89,106,124–128) describes any separation of the craniovertebral junction. The primary injury is ligamentous disruption and may result in complete (atlanto-occipital dislocation) or partial (atlanto-occipital subluxation) atlanto-occipital disassociation. The skull may be displaced anteriorly, posteriorly, cranially, or in a direction resulting from a combination of either anterior or posterior displacement with distraction.

Radiographically, atlanto-occipital disassociation may be manifested by displacement of the occipital condyles from the superior articulating facets of the atlas, a "Powers ratio" (129) greater than 1.0 (anterior dislocation only), or disruption of the normal relationship between the basion (tip of the clivus) and the tip of the dens (Fig. 3.20).

Atlantoaxial dislocation (Fig. 3.21) is usually associated with occipitoatlantal disassociation secondary to distraction.

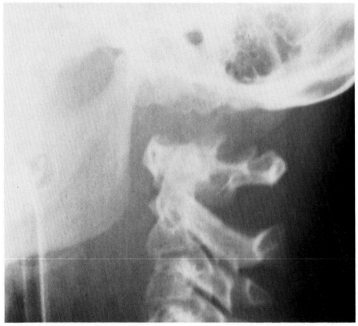

Figure 3.20. Longitudinal occipitoatlantal dislocation secondary to a distractive vector force. Enormous soft tissue swelling extends from the base of the skull throughout the cervical area.

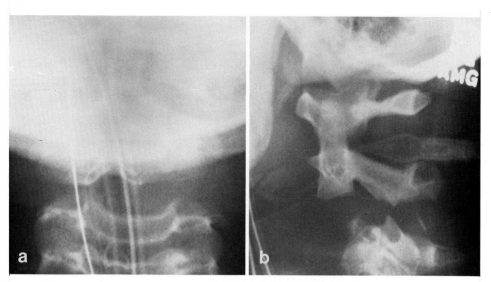

Figure 3.21. Atlantoaxial separation associated with distractive occipitoatlantal disassociation and C_2–C_3 disassociation seen in frontal (*a*) and lateral (*b*) projections.

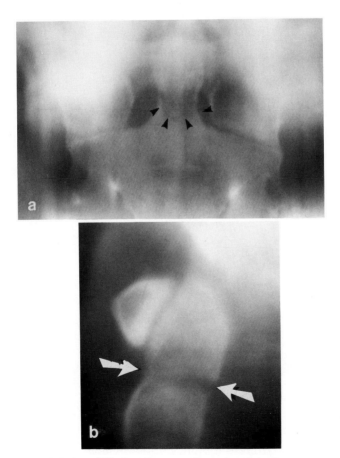

Figure 3.22. High (type II) dens fracture (*arrowheads*) in frontal (*a*) and lateral (*b*) tomograms.

Odontoid Fractures. These fractures have been described as resulting from "horizontal vector force from anterior to posterior transmitted through the skull to the dens" (98); "several complex forces, including flexion and extension and probably rotation" (130); "hyperflexion and hyperextension" (112); "hyperextension, direct force vector anterior to posterior causing shear failure, flexion, anterior translation" (18); "flexion, hyperextension, lateral hyperflexion" (62); and "lateral hyperflexion" (110).

Odontoid fractures have been classified by Anderson and D'Alonzo (131) as type I (avulsion fracture of the tip of the dens), type II

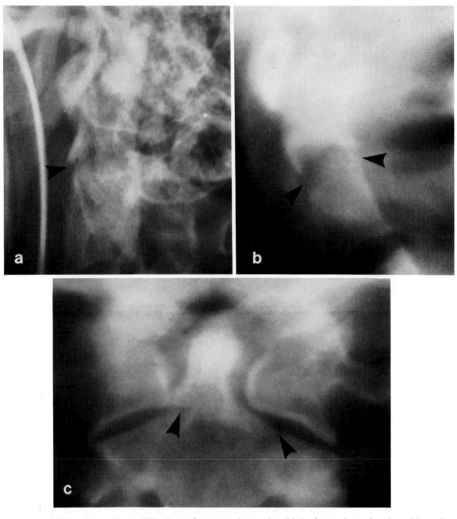

Figure 3.23. Low (type III) dens fracture (*arrowheads*) in lateral projection (*a*) and in lateral (*b*) and anteroposterior (*c*) tomograms. The axis "ring" is disrupted in the lateral projection.

(transverse fracture of the dens above the axis body) (Fig. 3.22), and type III (fracture of the superior portion of the axis body, which involves one or both superior articulating facets of the axis) (Fig. 3.23). The validity of a type I fracture has been challenged (51,99). If the type I fracture exists, it indicates occipitoatlantal disassociation, an entirely different connotation than the type II and III fractures that constitute atlantoaxial instability. Gehweiler, Osborne, and Becker (62) and Alexander and associates (132) have referred to the Anderson and D'Alonzo type II as "high" dens fractures and type III as "low" dens fractures. In lateral projection, the low dens fracture is distinguished from the high by disruption of the axis ring (133).

Chapter 4

Flexion Injuries

The mechanism of the flexion family of cervical spine injuries is pure or predominant acute hyperflexion. Selecki (51) and others (18,21,43,47,50,52,53,61) have demonstrated, experimentally, that the extent or type of cervical spine injury is directly related to the magnitude of the causative force, its direction, and the degree of flexion of the spine at the instant of injury. The same research has established that the most extensive flexion injury occurs following direct trauma to the head and neck in the flexed position, and that these injuries are characteristic and consist of the "drop" or "tear" fractures. Less severe flexion injuries probably occur when the spine is in a more neutral attitude and is driven into flexion by the vector force or by flexion forces of lesser magnitude.

ANTERIOR SUBLUXATION

(Hyperflexion Sprain)

Tear of the posterior ligament complex may occur as an isolated injury (anterior subluxation) or as an integral component of any cervical spine injury in which flexion is a major vector force.

Although Whitley and Forsyth (52) have described some of the roentgen signs of isolated anterior subluxation ("partial dislocation"), anterior subluxation of the cervical spine was a diagnosis commonly held in disrespect, if not frankly rejected, by most radiologists until precise and accurate descriptions of its radiographic signs (20,40,72) appeared in more recent literature. Braakman and Penning (134), referring to anterior subluxation as "hyperflexion sprain," prepared a classic and detailed description of this injury. Anterior subluxation was recognized by orthopaedists and neurosurgeons (51,64,69,71,74) and Stringa (73), Holdsworth (21), and Selecki (51) described the mechanism of injury and the pathophysiology of the lesion.

Cheshire (63) reported 21% delayed instability following anterior subluxation compared with 5–7% delayed instability associated with all other types of cervical injuries. It is currently estimated that as many as 50% of patients with anterior subluxation experience delayed instability. Jackson (69) cited the development of localized degenerative changes following anterior subluxation as evidence of soft tissue trauma at the time of injury.

Anterior subluxation is the result of a flexion force of less than 49 kg/cm^2 (51) which is the least amount of force capable of producing pathologic structural injury of the cervical spine (51).

The pathophysiology of anterior subluxation consists solely of disruption of the posterior ligament complex (the supra- and interspinous ligaments, the interfacetal joint capsules, the ligamentum flavum, and the posterior longitudinal ligament) (Fig. 4.1) (21, 51). The posterior portion of the annulus fibrosis and, to varying degrees, the posterior aspect of the intervertebral disk are torn while the majority of the disk, the anterior portion of the annulus and the anterior longitudinal ligament remain intact. This localized, posterior soft tissue disruption allows the vertebra immediately above the level of soft tissue injury to (*a*) rotate anteriorly, pivoting on its anterior inferior corner or (*b*) glide (translate) anteriorly with respect to the immediately subjacent vertebra. The pathology of anterior subluxation is schematically represented in Figures 4.2 and 4.3. Figure 4.2 represents subluxation in which the involved vertebra simply rotates anteriorly, pivoting on its anteroinferior corner. Figure 4.3 represents the concept of subluxation described by Holdsworth (21) in which there is frank but minimal (1–3 mm) anterior displacement of the vertebral body and subluxation, *but not frank dislocation*, of the interfacetal joints.

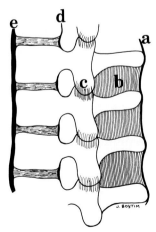

Figure 4.1. Schematic representation of the posterior ligament complex. *a*, supraspinous ligament; *b*, interspinous ligament; *c*, capsule of the facetal joint; *d*, posterior longitudinal ligament. The ligamentum flavum, an integral portion of the posterior ligament complex, is not shown. The anterior longitudinal ligament (*e*) is not part of the posterior ligament complex and is identified here for completeness.

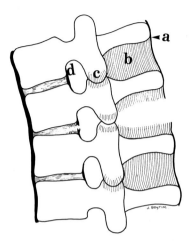

Figure 4.2. Schematic representation of the pathology of anterior subluxation without forward displacement of the subluxated vertebra. The posterior ligament complex (supraspinous ligament (*a*), interspinous ligament (*b*), facetal joint capsule (*c*), and posterior longitudinal ligament (*d*)) is disrupted and there is a short tear into the intervertebral disk. The anteroinferior corner of the vertebral body acts as the pivotal point for the anterior rotation of the involved segment, which results in the superior facet of the involved apophyseal joint gliding superiorly and anteriorly with respect to its contiguous inferior facet. (From Harris, J.H.,Jr.: Acute injuries of the spine. *Semin. Roentgenol.* 13:53, 1978.)

Because the skeletal stability provided by the normal anatomy of the interfacetal joints is maintained, although subluxated, and because the intervertebral disk is not completely disrupted and the anterior longitudinal ligament remains intact, anterior subluxation is initially stable.

The roentgen diagnosis of anterior subluxation may be very difficult because of the subtlety of the radiographic findings when the involved vertebra is not frankly anteriorly displaced and because some of the features of anterior subluxation may be simulated by voluntary (i.e., the "military" or the supine position (Fig. 4.4)) or involuntary (muscle spasm (Fig. 4.5)) straightening of the normal cervical lordosis. The physiologic changes in alignment of the cervical vertebrae due to positioning or muscle spasm may occur in either of two patterns: (*a*) the smooth, continuous, uninterrupted reversal of cervical lordosis or (*b*) reversal of cervical lordosis due to the progressively greater "step-wise" anterior translation (displacement) at each successively higher level (Fig. 4.5*a* and *b*). This concept is illustrated by comparing the alignment of the cervical vertebrae in Figures 1.17 (normal lateral), 1.24 (normal flexion), 4.5*a* (muscle spasm) and 4.6*a*, 4.7*a*, and 4.8*a* (anterior subluxation).

Careful evaluation of the lateral radiograph in neutral, flexion, and extension positions as well as strict adherence to the criteria of anterior subluxation are necessary to minimize "overreading." For

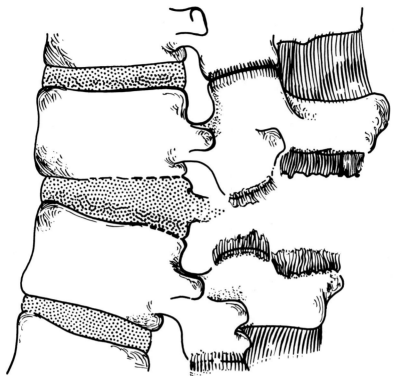

Figure 4.3. Schematic representation of the pathology of anterior subluxation as depicted by Holdsworth (8).

example, the patient illustrated in Figure 4.4 is a 16-year-old girl who was the passenger in an automobile that was struck from behind. She complained of severe, diffuse pain and moderate limitation of motion in the cervical area. There were no localizing neurologic signs or symptoms. In the neutral lateral radiograph (Fig. 4.4*a*), the normal cervical lordotic curve is reversed uniformly throughout the length of the cervical spine. The interspinous spaces are of similar width and the relationship of the articular facets and their contiguous posterior cortical margins are normal and uniform. To the degree that flexion and extension were possible, movement of the vertebral bodies and their posterior elements with respect to each other, was physiologic (Fig. 4.4*b* and *c*). Thus, although the patient sustained a flexion injury of the cervical spine, had pain and limitation of motion, and in the neutral lateral radiograph had *generalized, smooth, uninterrupted* reversal of the cervical lordosis, none of the criteria of anterior subluxation was present, even when the spine was "stressed" by flexion. Therefore, although this patient may have experienced a soft tissue injury in the cervical region, there is no radiographic evidence of anterior subluxation.

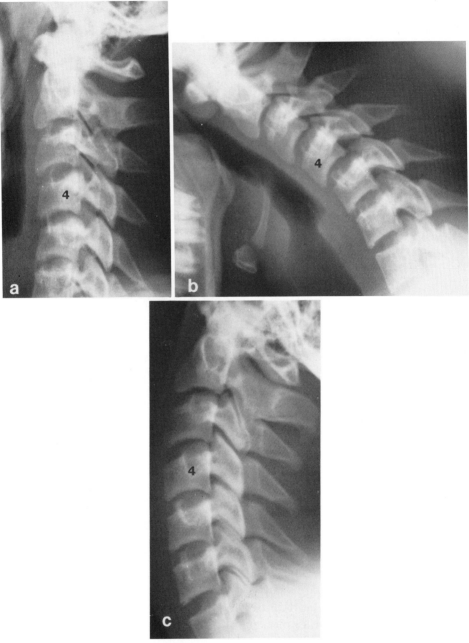

Figure 4.4. This patient was involved in a motor vehicle accident and complained of neck pain. The supine lateral radiograph (*a*) demonstrates an apparent hyperkyphotic angulation at the C_4–C_5 level, suggesting anterior subluxation. However, neither the interspinous nor the interlaminar spaces are widened, i.e., there is no "fanning," and the interfacetal joints are normal at this level. Specifically, the contiguous facets are parallel and their posterior margins are on the same vertical plane. Lateral flexion (*b*) and extension (*c*) radiographs demonstrate only physiologic motion of the cervical spine. Therefore, the posterior ligament complex at the C_4–C_5 level is intact, anterior subluxation is not present, and the appearance of the cervical spine in the supine lateral projection (*a*) is positional.

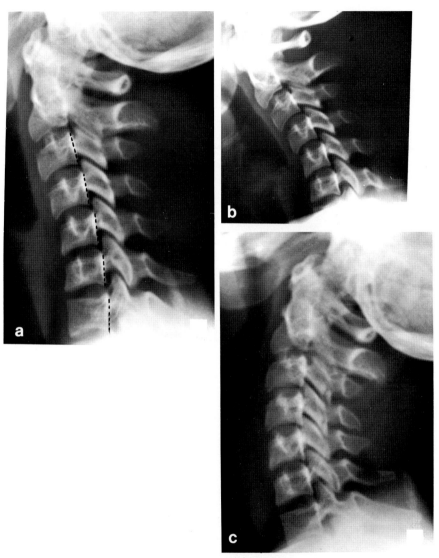

Figure 4.5. Lateral radiographs of the cervical spine made in neutral (*a*), flexion (*b*), and extension (*c*). This patient developed severe pain and limitation of motion of the neck following a rear-end automobile accident. The neutral lateral radiograph (*a*) demonstrates only smooth, continuous, uninterrupted diffuse reversal of the normal cervical lordosis. The interspinous spaces from C_3–C_7 are uniformly widened, the anatomy of the interfacetal joints is normal at each level, and each succeedingly higher vertebra has moved forward a slightly greater distance than the subjacent segment, resulting in the diffusely reversed curve. All of these findings are the result of muscle spasm. Lateral flexion (*b*) and extension (*c*) views record only the physiologic attitude of the cervical spine in those positions. This illustration emphasizes that even when the mechanism of injury and the clinical findings suggest anterior subluxation, the diagnosis rests not on simple reversal of the normal cervical lordosis, but on strict adherence to the radiographic criteria of anterior subluxation. This illustration should be compared with Figures 4.6–4.8, 4.12, and 4.13.

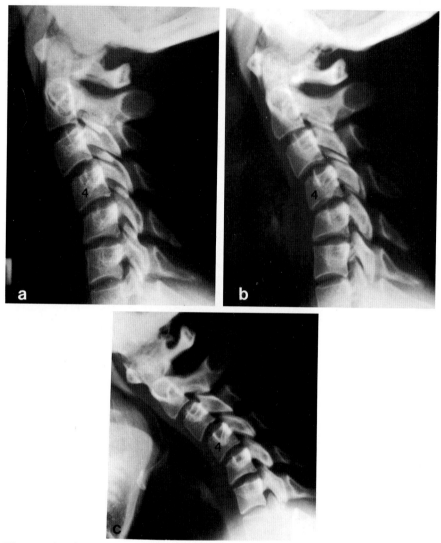

Figure 4.6.   (*a*) Anterior subluxation of C_4 on C_5 characterized by localized hyper-kyphotic angulation sustained at the time of initial injury. (*b*) Lateral neutral radiograph of the same patient several months later following minor trauma to the neck. The anterior subluxation persists. The lateral flexion radiograph (*c*) demonstrates and confirms, delayed instability. (From Grainger, R.C., and Allison, D.J.: *A Textbook of Organ Imaging.* New York, Churchill Livingstone, 1986, Chapter 68.)

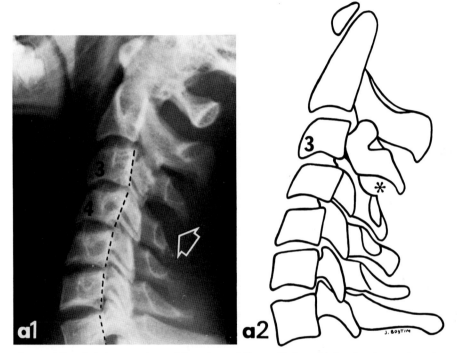

Figure 4.7. Subtle anterior subluxation of C_3 on C_4 in a high school wrestler who sustained a flexion injury. In the neutral lateral projection (*a1* and *a2*), there is a localized hyperkyphotic angulation at the C_3–C_4 level characterized by widening of the interspinous and interlaminar spaces (*open arrow*) and (*) subluxation of the interfacetal joints and narrowing of the intervertebral disk space anteriorly. In flexion (*b1* and *b2*), C_3 is clearly anteriorly displaced, causing the third interspace to become narrower anteriorly and wider posteriorly while the superior facets of the apophyseal joints at this level glide upward and forward on the inferior facets (*small open arrow*), and the interspinous space demonstrates greater fanning. In extension (*c1* and *c2*), all of the signs described in the neutral and flexion positions are reduced and the spine appears normal. (From Harris, J.H.,Jr. and Harris, W.H.: *The Radiology of Emergency Medicine.* Baltimore, Williams & Wilkins, 1975.)

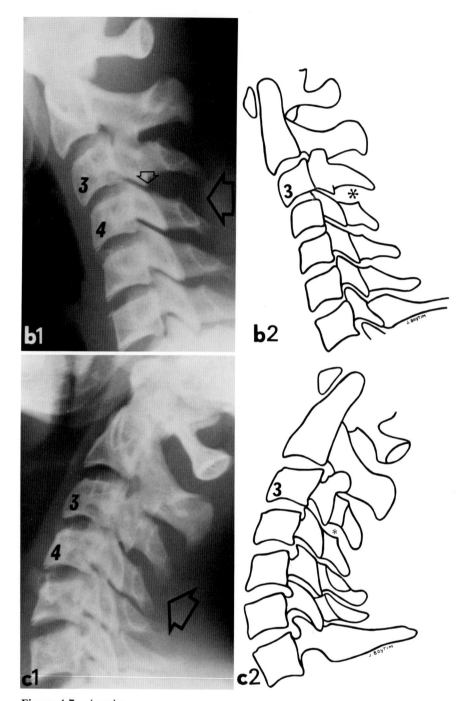

Figure 4.7.   *b* and *c.*

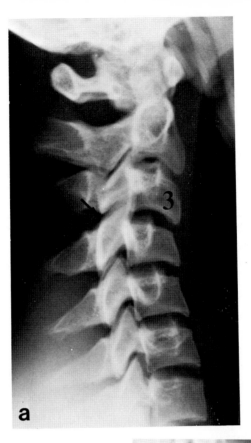

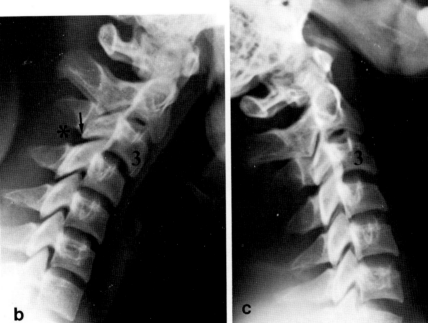

Figure 4.8. Anterior subluxation of C₃ on C₄. In the neutral (*a*) and flexion (*b*) lateral projections, the roentgen signs of anterior subluxation are clearly evident. These include anterior displacement of the body of C₃, anterior narrowing and posterior widening of the disk space, forward displacement of the superior facets of the apophyseal joints (*arrow*) and fanning (*). In sum, these changes all constitute the localized hyperkyphotic angulation of anterior subluxation. The relationship of the facets of the subluxated apophyseal joints is well demonstrated, particularly when compared with the facetal joints at the lower levels. In extension (*c*), all of the signs of anterior subluxation are reversed and the spine appears normal.

The clinical condition of the patient is extremely important in the evaluation of the radiographs. Patients with acute anterior subluxation typically have severe pain, marked limitation of flexion and extension, and point tenderness over the involved interspinous spaces.

"Delayed instability" (63) of previous anterior subluxation is *relatively* pain free and is not characterized by marked limitation of motion. This concept is illustrated by the patient in Figure 4.6 who sustained an acute anterior subluxation of C_4–C_5 (Fig. 4.6a) that was associated with severe pain and marked limitation of motion, as the result of an automobile accident. Several months later, the patient fell a short distance, striking her head, neck, and shoulder on soft ground. She had minimal discomfort and no limitation of motion. The roentgen examination following the second accident demonstrated the original anterior subluxation with its persistent deformity and instability (Fig. 4.6b).

Radiographically, the cardinal feature of anterior subluxation that distinguishes it from the physiologic attitude of the cervical spine in the straight ("military") or flexed position is an abrupt change in cervical lordosis characterized by localized hyperkyphotic angulation limited to the level(s) of posterior ligament tear (Figs. 4.6–4.9) (20).

> *In the following discussion, the term "superior facet" refers to the superior facet of the interfacetal (apophyseal) joint, i.e., the inferior facet of the vertebra above, and "inferior facet" (of the joint) refers to the superior facet of the vertebra below.*

At the level of subluxation, the interspinous and interlaminar spaces are abnormally wide as a result of disruption of the supraspinous and interspinous ligaments. Increase in width of the interspinous space has been called "fanning" (66). The superior facets of the apophyseal joints are displaced upward and forward with respect to their contiguous inferior facets. This movement of the superior facets is evidenced by the increased distance between the posterior cortical margins of the contiguous facets at the level of subluxation (Fig. 4.9) in comparison to that of the uninvolved levels. Although the superior facets are subluxated (partially dislocated), they maintain their normal posterior position relative to the subjacent inferior facets of the joint. The intervertebral disk space becomes widened posteriorly and narrowed anteriorly as a result of forward rotation of the involved vertebral body. The involved vertebra may or may not be displaced anteriorly with respect to the subjacent vertebra (Fig. 4.9).

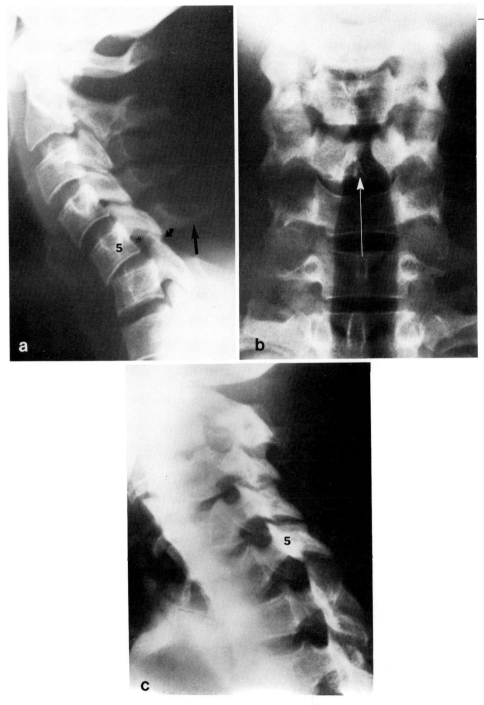

Figure 4.9. Anterior subluxation of C_5 on C_6. As a result of the anterior translation and rotation of C_5, the lateral radiograph (*a*) demonstrates localized hyperkyphosis at this level, anterior narrowing and posterior widening of the intervertebral disk, separation of the posterior cortex of the vertebral body of C_5 from that of the anterior cortex of the subjacent articular mass (*). subluxation of the interfacetal joints (*curved arrow*) and widening of the interlaminar and interspinous spaces ("fanning") (*long arrow*). These are the characteristic radiographic signs of anterior subluxation. In the frontal projection (*b*), the C_5–C_6 spinous space is abnormally widened (*arrow*), reflecting distraction of the posterior column and "fanning" associated with tear of the posterior ligament complex. The oblique projection (*c*) demonstrates the incomplete dislocation (subluxation) of the left articular mass of C_5 with respect to that of C_6.

The radiographic signs of anterior subluxation have been summarized as (*a*) a localized kyphotic angulation at the level of injury; (*b*) anterior rotation, with or without displacement, of the subluxated vertebra; (*c*) anterior narrowing and posterior widening of the disk space; (*d*) widening of the space between the subluxed vertebral body and the subjacent articular masses; (*e*) displacement of the inferior articulating facets of the subluxated vertebra with respect to their contiguous subjacent facets; and (*f*) widening of the interspinous or interlaminar space ("fanning") (20).

Widening of the interspinous distance ("fanning") in the *anteroposterior* radiograph of the lower cervical spine is an important sign of a flexion injury, including anterior subluxation. The increased interspinous distance confirms subtle "fanning" on the lateral radiograph (Fig. 4.10) or may indicate posterior ligamentous tear when, on the lateral radiograph of the cervical spine, the involved segments are obscured by the density of the shoulders (Fig. 4.11).

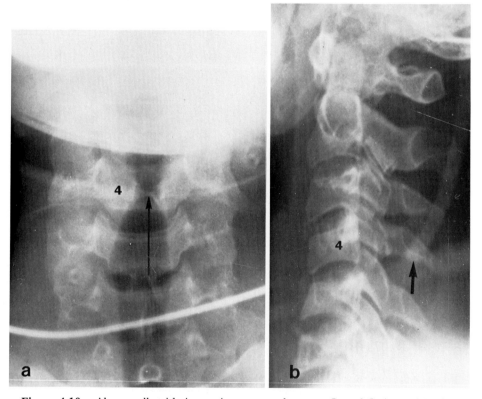

Figure 4.10. Abnormally wide interspinous space between C₄ and C₅ (*arrows*) in the frontal projection (*a*) indicates the "fanning" and disruption of the posterior ligament complex seen in the lateral projection (*b*). In the lateral radiograph, localized hyperkyphosis at the C₄–C₅ level, anterior rotation *without* translation of C₄, anterior narrowing and posterior widening of the intervertebral disk, and subluxation of the interfacetal joints are also evident.

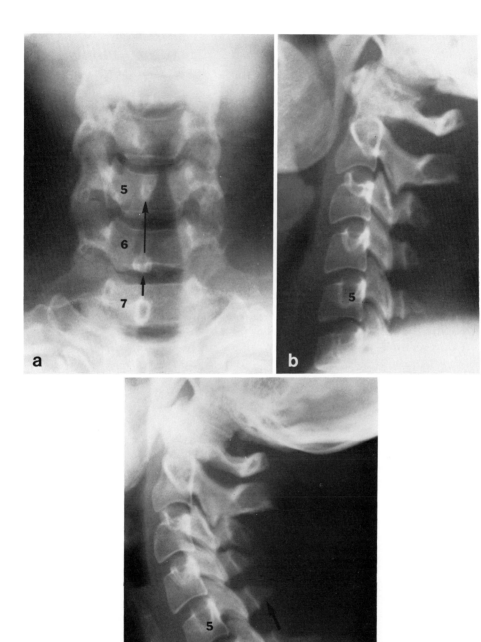

Figure 4.11. Increase in the C_5–C_6 and, to a lesser degree, the C_6–C_7 interspinous distances (*arrow*) in the frontal projection (*a*) reflects a posterior ligament complex tear that is not visible on the initial lateral radiograph (*b*) because of the superimposed density of the shoulders. In a subsequent lateral radiograph (*c*) in which the lower cervical segments are well seen, anterior subluxation at the C_5–C_6 level and, to a lesser degree, at the C_6–C_7 level is confirmed.

All of the roentgen signs of anterior subluxation are accentuated in flexion and reduced in extension.

The roentgen signs of delayed or failed ligamentous healing ("delayed instability") are seen in Figures 4.12 and 4.13. The morbidity of "delayed instability" is sufficient to warrant emphasizing, by repetition, that (a) "delayed instability" is commonly a complication of "minor" acute cervical spine injuries, i.e., anterior subluxation or "simple" wedge fracture and (b) the incidence of "delayed instability" following subluxation ranges from 21–50% (63).

Anterior subluxation usually occurs at a single level but, depending on the magnitude and direction of the causative force, may involve more than one cervical segment (Figs. 4.11 and 4.14). In recumbency, anterior subluxation may be even more difficult to identify than usual and may be heralded only by an inappropriate interspinous distance ("fanning"). If the supine lateral radiograph is suggestive of anterior subluxation, or is equivocal, a lateral examination made in flexion—even recumbent if dictated by the clinical circumstances—should establish the diagnosis (Fig. 4.15). When anterior subluxation occurs

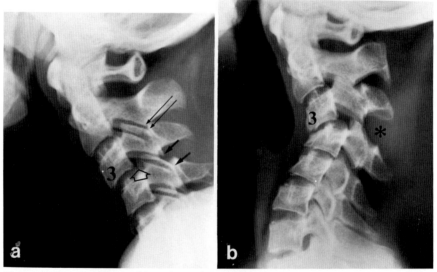

Figure 4.12. Anterior subluxation of C_3 on C_4. In the neutral lateral radiograph made at the time of acute injury (a), the forward displacement of C_3 is obvious. Since the entire vertebra is anteriorly subluxated, the space between the posterior cortex of the body of C_3 and the anterior cortex of the articular masses of C_4 has increased (*open arrow*) and the superior facet of the involved apophyseal joint has moved forward on its inferior facet. The *short arrows* indicate the distance between the posterior margins of the articular facets of one apophyseal joint at the level of subluxation. The *long arrows* indicate this distance at a normal apophyseal joint. The neutral lateral radiograph (b) of the same patient 8 months later demonstrated severe delayed instability with marked fanning (*). (From Harris, J. H., Jr.: Acute injuries of the spine. *Semin. Roentgenol.* 13:53, 1978.)

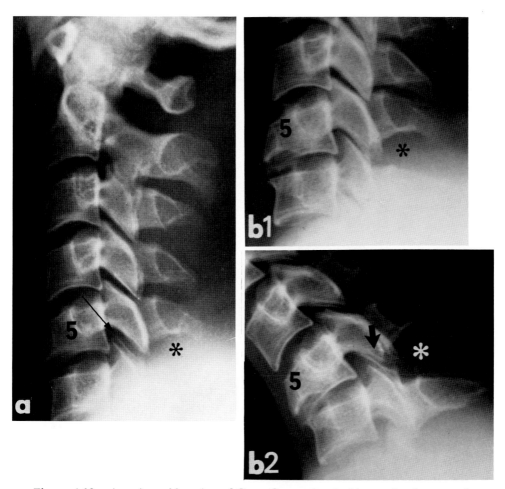

Figure 4.13. Anterior subluxation of C_5 on C_6 associated with a wedge fracture of C_5. Although the wedge fracture is the most striking abnormality, some of the signs of anterior subluxation are evident (*a*). The fifth vertebra is slightly anteriorly displaced and rotated on its inferior corner, the C_5–C_6 interfacetal joint space is widened (*arrow*) and, even though incompletely visualized, the interspinous space appears widened (*). Lateral neutral (*b1*) and flexion (*b2*) views made 18 months after the original injury indicate the delayed instability at this level by the abnormal forward displacement of C_5 in flexion (*b2*). The interspinous space is widened (*), the inferior facets of C_5 are displaced forward (*b2, arrow*), and the disk space is widened posteriorly and narrowed anteriorly.

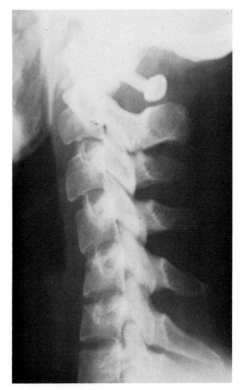

Figure 4.14.   Anterior subluxation at the C_4–C_5 and C_5–C_6 levels.

in conjunction with degenerative disease of the cervical spine, it usually occurs in the uninvolved levels (Fig. 4.16).

Although anterior subluxation is a discrete injury, the posterior ligament complex is disrupted as an integral component of other flexion injuries. When associated with the "simple" wedge fracture (Figs. 4.17 and 4.18), the posterior ligament complex tear may be the more significant lesion leading to "delayed instability" (63) secondary to failure of ligamentous healing (20) (Fig. 4.13). Disruption of the posterior ligament complex is an integral, but relatively insignificant, component of the total ligamentous disruption that occurs in both bilateral interfacetal dislocation (BID) and the flexion teardrop fracture. Conversely, the *intact* posterior ligament complex is the basis for the avulsion fracture of a cervicothoracic spinous process (clay shoveler's fracture).

The posterior ligament complex is disrupted in unilateral interfacetal dislocation (UID) caused by simultaneous flexion and rotation, but remains intact in cervical spine injuries with a hyperextension mechanism of injury.

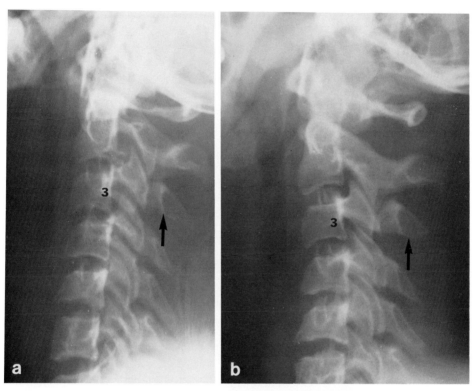

Figure 4.15. The most prominent sign of anterior subluxation in the initial supine lateral radiograph (*a*) is "fanning" at the C₃–C₄ level. A subtle, but definite, localized hyperkyphotic angulation is present at this level as well. Because the changes of anterior subluxation in the initial supine lateral radiograph were so subtle, a supine flexion lateral examination (*b*) was obtained by placing a sandbag under the occiput. This examination demonstrates all the radiographic signs of anterior subluxation, including "fanning" (*arrow*), and confirms the diagnosis.

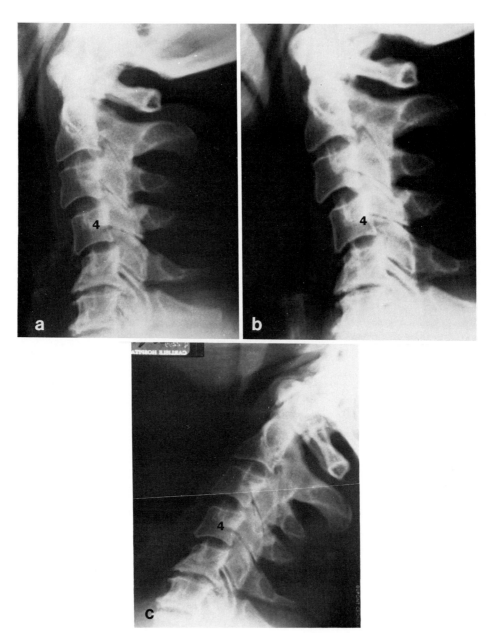

Figure 4.16.   Anterior subluxation of C_4 on C_5 in a patient with degenerative disease of the lower cervical spine in the neutral (*a*) and flexed (*b*) lateral projections. In the extension lateral radiograph (*c*) the signs of anterior subluxation are reduced, which is characteristic of this injury.

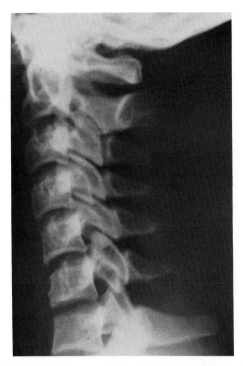

Figure 4.17. Simple wedge fracture of C_6 evidenced by a slight decrease in anterior height of the vertebral body and disruption and impaction of its anterior cortex. All signs of anterior subluxation are also present at this level, including localized hyper-kyphosis, "fanning," subluxation of facetal joints, and increase in the distance between the body of C_6 and the articular masses of C_7.

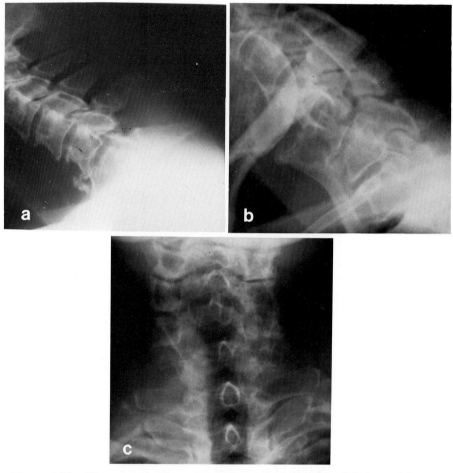

Figure 4.18. The acute simple wedge (compression) fracture of C₇ is partially seen in the lateral radiograph (*a*) and more completely demonstrated in the "swimmer's" view (*b*). Signs of disruption of the posterior ligament complex and of anterior subluxation are clearly evident in the lateral radiograph (*a*) and in the frontal projection (*c*) by widening of the interspinous space at C₆–C₇.

BILATERAL INTERFACETAL DISLOCATION (BID)

The majority of authors believe that BID is the result of hyperflexion injury (52,102,100,66,134,48) "very close to the sagittal plane." (18) Others (21,63,50,54) contend that BID results from combined flexion and rotational forces. It is appropriate to consider bilateral interfacetal dislocation as a flexion injury because BID has been experimentally produced by a flexion mechanism, because the roentgen appearance of bilateral interfacetal dislocation contains very little or no intimation of a rotational component, and because BID is reduced by straight traction. Both unilateral and bilateral interfacetal dislocations are primarily soft tissue injuries with posterior ligament complex tear common to each. In BID, the intervertebral disk and anterior longitudinal ligament are disrupted as well.

The pathophysiology of bilateral interfacetal dislocation includes complete disruption of the posterior ligament complex, the posterior longitudinal ligament, the intervertebral disk, usually the anterior longitudinal ligament (43,135), and anterior dislocation of the superior facets (and, obviously, their articular masses) of the interfacetal joint with respect to the inferior facets at the level of injury. The dislocated facets pass upward, forward, and over the inferior facets of the joint, coming to rest in the intervertebral foramina.

Bilateral interfacetal dislocation may be partial or complete. When the dislocation is incomplete, the dislocated vertebra is anteriorly displaced a distance somewhat less than one-half the anteroposterior diameter of the vertebral body. The posteroinferior margins of the inferior facets of the dislocated vertebra may come to rest astride the anterosuperior margins of the superior facets of the subjacent vertebra ("perched" vertebra) (Fig. 4.19) or the dislocated articular masses may sit high in the intervertebral foramina (Figs. 4.20a and 4.21a).

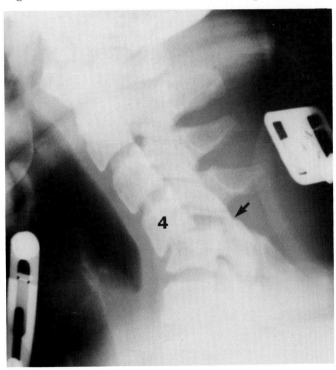

Figure 4.19. Incomplete BID ("perched" vertebra). C_4 is translated anteriorly in flexion with respect to C_5 to the degree that the posterior margin of the inferior facets of C_4 sit atop the anterior margins of the superior facets of C_5 (*arrow*). This amount of displacement and disruption of the interfacetal joints is greater than occurs in partial dislocation (anterior subluxation), but less than in frank bilateral interfacetal dislocation in which each articular mass of the dislocated vertebra is situated completely anterior to its subjacent counterpart.

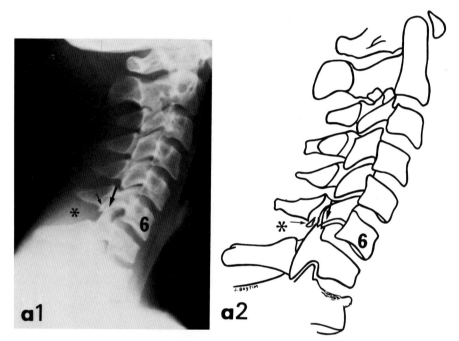

Figure 4.20. Incomplete bilateral interfacetal dislocation. In the lateral radiograph (*a1* and *a2*), the dislocated sixth segment is anteriorly displaced. The superior facet of each apophyseal joint (*large arrow*) appears to be "perched" upon its contiguous inferior facet. A tiny fragment remains posterior to the inferior facet (*small arrow*). The interspinous space is abnormally wide (*). Incidental wedge fractures involve the bodies of C_7 and T_1. The oblique projections (*b1* and *b2* and *c1* and *c2*) confirm that on each side, the dislocated superior facet of the joint (*arrow*) lies just anterior to the subjacent articular mass and within the intervertebral foramen. (From Harris, J. H., Jr.: Acute injuries of the spine. *Semin. Roentgenol.* 13:53, 1978.)

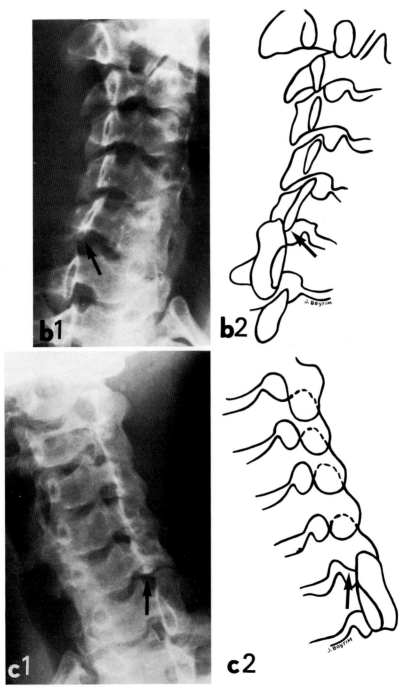

Figure 4.20. *b* and *c.*

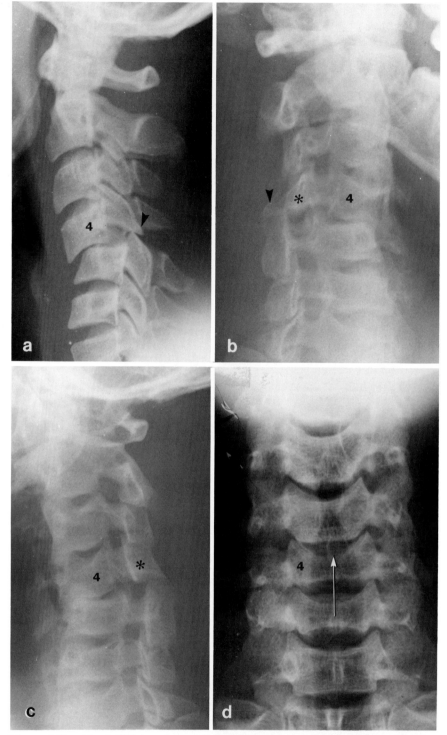

Figure 4.21. Frank BID is only established in this patient in the oblique projections (*b* and *c*). On the right (*b*), the articular mass of C₄ (∗) lies clearly in the intervertebral foramen. A small fracture fragment (*arrowhead*) arises from the posterolateral aspect of the inferior portion of the right articular mass of C₄. On the left (*c*), the articular mass of C₄ (∗) is situated high in the intervertebral foramen. In the lateral radiograph (*a*), although the body of C₄ is anteriorly translated approximately 50% of the antero-posterior diameter of the body, the articular masses do not appear to be completely dislocated. The small fracture fragment seen in the right anterior oblique (*b*) projection is also evident in the lateral (*arrowhead*) radiograph. In the frontal projection (*d*), the C₄–C₅ interspinous space (*arrow*) is abnormally wide.

Oblique radiographs are essential to establish the degree and bilaterality of incomplete bilateral interfacetal dislocation (Figs. 4.20*b* and *c* and 4.21*b* and *c*).

Beatson (43) has demonstrated experimentally that *complete* bilateral interfacetal dislocation can occur only with total disruption of the posterior ligament complex, the intervertebral disk, and the anterior longitudinal ligament. Because of these skeletal derangements and soft tissue injuries, the dislocated vertebra is anteriorly displaced a distance equivalent to one-half of the anteroposterior diameter, or greater, of the vertebral body (Figs. 4.22–4.24). These cadaver experiments have established that it is impossible for frank bilateral interfacetal dislocation to occur without this magnitude of displacement of the vertebral body. Consequently, when this degree of anterior displacement of the vertebral body is seen in the lateral radiograph, it is characteristic of bilateral interfacetal dislocation, and oblique radiographs are not required to establish the diagnosis.

In the anteroposterior radiograph of the cervical spine, BID is characterized by all of the spinous processes being in the midline and

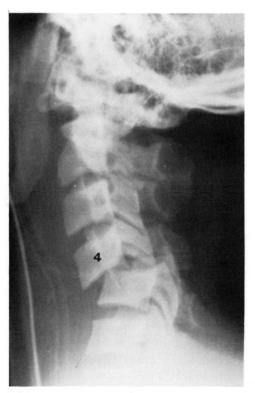

Figure 4.22. Frank, complete BID. Each articular mass of C$_4$ is completely anteriorly displaced with respect to those of C$_5$. (From Grainger, R.C. and Allison, D.J.: *A Textbook of Organ Imaging*. New York, Churchill Livingstone, 1968, Chapter 68.)

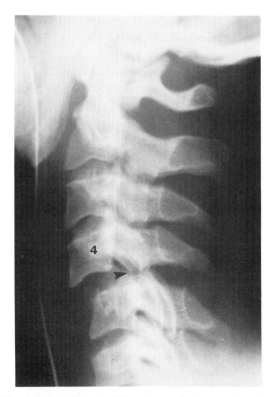

Figure 4.23. Bilateral interfacetal dislocation. C_4 is translated anteriorly to the degree that approximately 50% of its vertebral body is anterior to that of C_5. The intervertebral disk space is abnormally wide. The inferior facets of C_4 each lie anterior to the subjacent facets of C_5. The posterior cortex of at least one of the inferior facets of C_4 is fractured (*arrowhead*).

an increased interspinous distance at the level of the dislocation (Fig. 4.21*d*).

Frequently, a small impaction fracture that may arise from the posterior margin of the inferior facet of the dislocated vertebra or from the anterior margin of the superior facet of the subjacent vertebra can be demonstrated radiographically (Figs. 4.20*a* and 4.21*a*). Bedbrook (136) verified the presence of such fractures in each of 70 patients with bilateral interfacetal dislocation examined at autopsy or surgical exploration. In Bedbrook's series, these fractures were commonly not visible radiographically (Fig. 4.23). In view of the extensive soft tissue injury associated with BID, however, these fractures are considered to be of relatively little clinical significance.

Bilateral interfacetal dislocation, because of its extensive soft tissue damage and dislocated facetal joints, is unstable and is associated with a high incidence of cord damage (18,41,43,48,74,135,137).

Bilateral interfacetal dislocation is occasionally referred to as "the double locked vertebra," "locked facets" (138), or "interlocking of

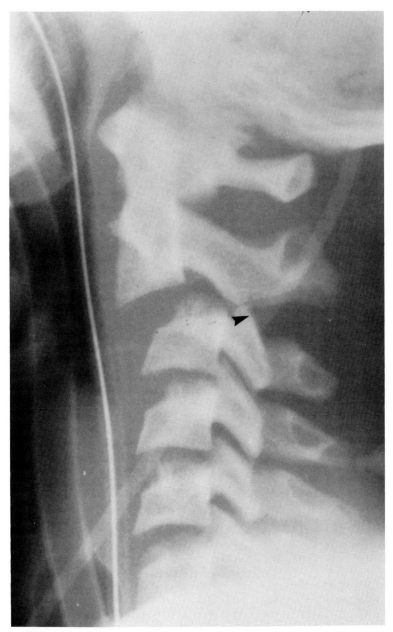

Figure 4.24. Complete, frank BID with each articular mass of C$_2$ displaced completely anteriorly with respect to those of C$_3$. The posterior margins of the inferior facets of C$_2$ are clearly seen to lie anterior to the anterior margins of the superior facets of C$_3$ (*arrowhead*).

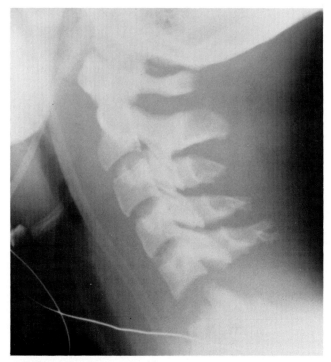

Figure 4.25.   Distracted BID with marked, diffuse prevertebral soft tissue swelling.

articular facets" (139), presumably because, on each side, the articular mass of the dislocated vertebra is seated within the inferior portion of the intervertebral foramen, as in the stable UID ("locked" vertebra). The implication, then, is that bilateral interfacetal dislocation, an inherently unstable injury, is mechanically stable when nothing could be further from the truth. For this reason, any use of the word "locked" in reference to bilateral interfacetal dislocation is pathologically inaccurate, clinically misleading, and should be avoided. The concept of the instability of BID secondary to ligamentous disruption and interfacetal joint dislocation is exquisitely illustrated in Figure 4.25.

WEDGE FRACTURE

("Simple" Wedge, "Simple" Compression Fracture)

A flexion force greater than that which causes an isolated anterior subluxation results in the "simple" wedge fracture of a vertebral body (18,51), which generally occurs in the mid or lower cervical segments (Fig. 4.26c). The mechanism of injury of the wedge fracture is mechanical compression of the involved centrum between the adjacent vertebral bodies.

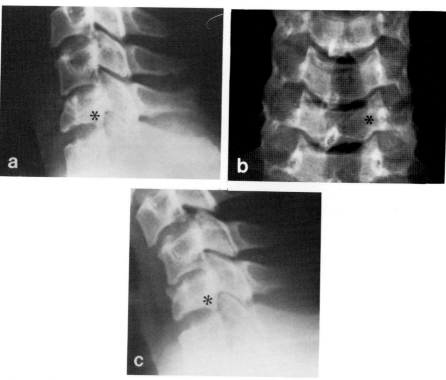

Figure 4.26. Simple wedge compression fracture of C_6 (*). In the neutral lateral projection (*a*), the vertebral body is decreased in stature anteriorly and both its superior end-plate and anterior cortex are buckled. In the frontal projection (*b*), the vertical body of C_6 (*) is diminished in vertical height but no fracture is visible. The flexion lateral radiograph (*c*) obtained several months after the initial injury demonstrates the impaction and compression of the body of C_6 by that of C_5 that occurred during hyperflexion at the time of the acute injury. Minor but definite soft tissue swelling is present throughout the lower cervical spine.

The posterior ligament complex may remain intact or be partially or completely disrupted as in anterior subluxation. Because the intervertebral disk and both the anterior and posterior longitudinal ligaments usually remain intact and because the structural integrity of the interfacetal joints is normally maintained, the wedge fracture is initially stable. However, in the event of concomitant posterior ligament complex tear, failure of the posterior ligament complex to heal may result in "delayed" instability, even though the wedge fracture heals (Figs. 4.12 and 4.13). In that event, the soft tissue injury is the principal lesion.

In the lateral radiograph, the simple wedge fracture is most commonly characterized by anterior loss of stature of the involved vertebral body, by impaction ("buckling," "step-off") of its anterior cortex and/or by disruption of the superior end-plate (Fig. 4.27). A thin, horizontal band of increased density representing impacted trabeculae

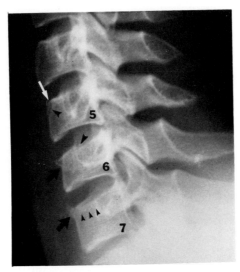

Figure 4.27.   Simple wedge fractures of the lower cervical vertebrae. An oblique, minimally displaced fracture involves the anterosuperior corner (*arrowhead*) of the centrum of C_5 with very slight but definite compression of the extreme anterior aspect of its superior end-plate (*top arrow*). There is anterior loss of stature of the body of C_6 secondary to the compression fracture involving its superior end-plate (*arrowhead*) and extending to, and causing buckling of, its anterior cortex (*arrow*). The anterosuperior cortex of C_7 is disrupted (*arrow*) and a thin, faint, dense band (*three small arrowheads*) beneath and parallel to its superior end-plate represents impacted trabeculae. (From Harris, J.H., Jr. and Harris, W.H.: *The Radiology of Emergency Medicine*, ed 2. Baltimore, Williams & Wilkins, 1981.)

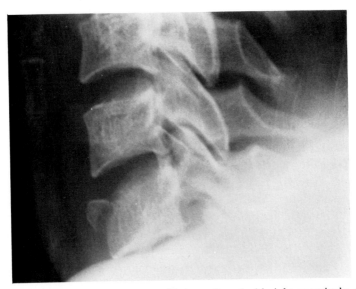

Figure 4.28.   Simple wedge fracture with loss of vertical height anteriorly, compression of the superior end-plate and a separate fragment comprised in the anterior superior corner of the involved vertebra. Minor, localized soft tissue swelling is present. In this projection, it is impossible to evaluate the integrity of the posterior ligament complex at this level, although it could reasonably be presumed to be torn based upon the characteristics of the fracture.

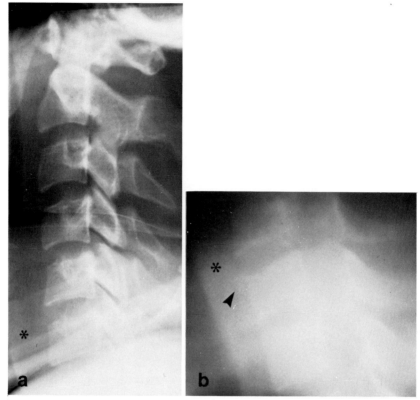

Figure 4.29. The simple wedge fracture of C_7 is obscured in the lateral plain radiograph (*a*) of the cervical spine because of the density of the superimposed shadows and is seen only by polydirectional tomography (*b*). The fracture is characterized by compression of the superior end-plate of the vertebral body, anterior loss of vertical height, and a separate displaced fragment (*arrowhead*) that consists of the anterosuperior corner of the vertebral body. Localized soft tissue swelling (*) is seen in both the plain-film and the tomogram.

may extend through the anteroposterior diameter of the vertebral body subjacent to the superior end-plate. With flexion force of greater magnitude, the anterosuperior corner of the vertebral body may constitute a separate fragment (Figs. 4.28 and 4.29). When present, prevertebral soft tissue swelling is usually minimal and localized to the area of the involved segment (Fig. 4.26). In the anteroposterior projection, the involved vertebra may be of normal or decreased stature (Fig. 4.26). The absence of a vertical fracture of the vertebral body with a wedge fracture helps to distinguish the wedge fracture from the burst fracture caused by axial loading (vertical compression).

CLAY SHOVELER'S FRACTURE

The clay shoveler's fracture, also called "coal miner's" fracture, "shoveler's disease," or "shoveler's" fracture, is an avulsion fracture of the spinous process of C_7, C_6, or T_1, in that order of frequency. This injury

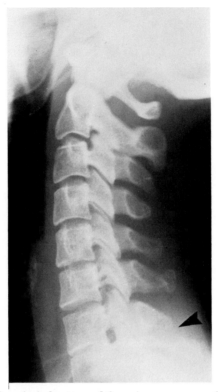

Figure 4.30.   Clay shoveler's fracture of the spinous process of C$_7$ (*arrowhead*). (From Harris, J.H., Jr. and Harris, W.H.: *The Radiology of Emergency Medicine.* Baltimore, Williams & Wilkins, 1975.)

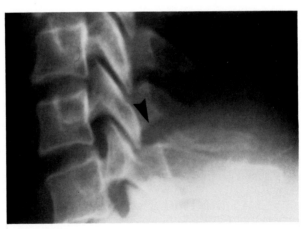

Figure 4.31.   Atypical clay shoveler's fracture in which the fracture line extends beyond the spinous process into the lamina (*arrowhead*). The typical clay shoveler's fracture, being limited to the spinous process, does not involve the spinal canal. The fracture illustrated does, raising the possibility of spinal cord injury.

is the result of an abrupt flexion of the head and neck against the tense "set" of the posterior ligaments, resulting in an oblique fracture typically limited to the proximal portion of the spinous process (Fig. 4.30). As is characteristic of all avulsion fractures, the fracture line is perpendicular to the orientation of the fibers of the interspinous ligament through which the causative vector force is mediated. Atypically, the fracture may extend to the lamina (Fig. 4.31), thereby involving the spinal canal with the potential of spinal cord injury. The clay shoveler's fracture is stable.

FLEXION TEARDROP FRACTURE

The most severe flexion force produces the "flexion teardrop fracture," which is the most devastating injury of the cervical spine compatible with life. This lesion, described by Schneider and Kahn in 1956 (85), derives its name from the characteristic triangle-shaped separate fragment that comprises the anteroinferior corner of the vertebral body. This fragment has been likened to a tear falling from a cheek.

Clinically, the flexion teardrop fracture is characterized by the "acute anterior cervical cord syndrome" (86, 140). This syndrome consists of immediate complete quadriplegia with loss of pain, temperature, and touch sensations (anterior column senses) and retention of the posterior column senses of position, motion, and vibration.

Pathologically, the anterior longitudinal ligament, the intervertebral disk, and the posterior longitudinal ligament are all disrupted. The reciprocal distractive force that occurs in the posterior column of the spine results in disruption of the posterior ligament complex and either subluxation or frank dislocation of the interfacet joints. Thus, there is neither ligamentous nor skeletal stability at the level of the injury and the flexion teardrop fracture is completely unstable.

Radiographically, in the lateral projection the attitude of the cervical spine is that of flexion from the level of the injury upward. The vertebral body fracture consists of a major separate triangular fragment comprising the anteroinferior corner of the body—the "teardrop" fragment. Although other tiny fragments may be present at the major fracture site, the centrum is not severely comminuted as is characteristic of the "bursting" fracture of the lower cervical spine. The spinal canal is narrowed at the level of injury by posterior angulation of the anterior column secondary to posterior displacement of the involved vertebral body. Consequently, the spinal canal is severely compromised. The involved vertebra is displaced and rotated anteriorly, and the interfacet joints are either bilaterally subluxated or dislocated. Disruption of the posterior ligament complex is evidenced by "fanning" (widening of the interlaminar and interspinous spaces) (Figs. 4.32–4.34).

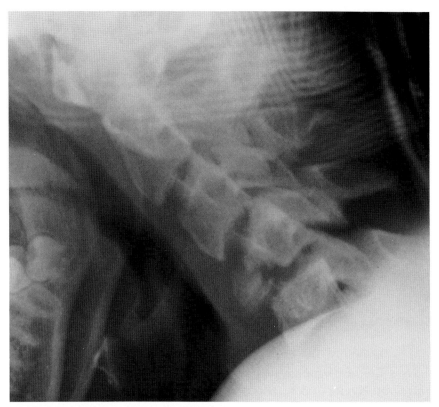

Figure 4.32.   Flexion teardrop fracture of C_4. The spine is flexed above the level of the injury and marked posterior angulation is present at this level. The triangle-shaped anterior fragment is displaced anteriorly, resulting in the characteristic teardrop configuration. The fragmentation and retropulsion of the vertebral body indicate that the anterior longitudinal ligament, the intervertebral disk, and the posterior longitudinal ligament are disrupted. Posteriorly, the interfacetal joints are subluxated and the interspinous space is widened, indicating disruption of the posterior ligament complex. (From Harris, J.H., Jr.: Acute injuries of the spine. *Semin. Roentgenol.* 13:53, 1978.)

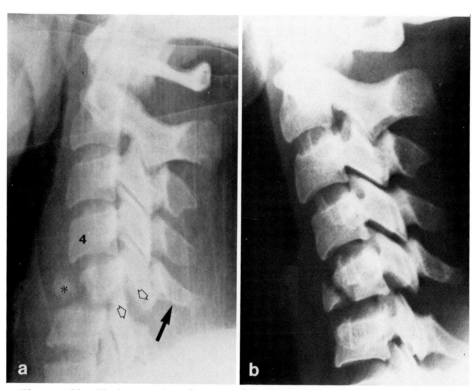

Figure 4.33. Flexion teardrop fracture of C₅. The initial supine lateral radiograph demonstrates a severe kyphotic deformity at the C₅–C₆ level. Compression of the anterior column of the spine has produced the characteristic large triangular fragment that comprises the anteroinferior aspect of the majority of the body of C₅ (*). Concomitant and reciprocal distraction of the posterior column is evidenced by disruption of the interfacetal joints (*open arrows*) and the interlaminar and interspinous spaces ("fanning") (*long arrow*). Marked diffuse prevertebral soft tissue swelling in the lower cervical spine indicates hemorrhage and edema. A subsequent lateral radiograph (*b*) demonstrates the characteristics of the teardrop fragment more clearly, as well as the flexion attitude of the upper cervical segments and total ligamentous disruption at the level of injury.

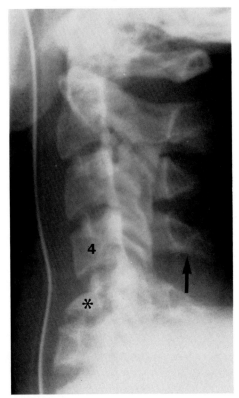

Figure 4.34. Flexion teardrop fracture of C_5 demonstrating the acute flexion deformity at the C_4–C_5 level, the large triangular fragment comprising the anteroinferior corner of the body of C_5 (∗), retropulsion of the remainder of the C_5 body fragment, anterior rotation and translation of C_4, subluxation of the C_4–C_5 interfacetal joints, and "fanning" of the C_4–C_5 interlaminar and interspinous processes (*arrow*). These are the signs of severe hyperflexion that, together with the characteristic fracture of the body of C_5, constitute the flexion teardrop fracture.

Correct identification of and distinction between the flexion teardrop fracture and the burst (vertical compression, "bursting," dispersion, axial loading) fracture of the lower cervical spine are of fundamental clinical importance because of the significant difference in neurologic involvement, stability, and management of these injuries. The flexion teardrop fracture is caused by severe flexion (84), has a typical radiographic appearance, is completely unstable, and is by definition associated with the acute anterior cervical cord syndrome, including permanent quadriplegia. The burst fracture, on the other hand, is caused by a vertical compression (axial loading) mechanism of injury directed through the straightened cervical spine, is characterized by comminution of the vertebral body, and is stable. Although posterior fragments may impinge upon the cord (41), neurologic involvement with the burst fracture depends on the extent and type of cord damage with the neurologic deficit ranging from transient paresthesia to permanent quadriplegia.

Chapter 5

Simultaneous Hyperflexion and Rotation: Unilateral Interfacetal Dislocation

Whereas pure, or dominant, flexion force produces a family of acute cervical spine injuries, including bilateral interfacetal dislocation, simultaneous flexion and rotation mechanism produce only the unilateral interfacetal dislocation (UID). An interfacetal joint on the side of the direction of rotation acts as the pivotal point while the articular mass of the contralateral side including its inferior facet (which is the superior facet of the interfacetal joint) rides upward, forward, and over the tip of the superior facet of the subjacent vertebra (the inferior facet of the involved joint) and comes to rest in the intervertebral foramen anterior to the superior articular mass (Fig. 5.1). In this position, the dislocated facet (and its articular mass) is mechanically "locked" (88) in place between the subjacent articular mass posteriorly and the vertebral body anteriorly. Because of the fixed position of the dislocated facet (and articular mass), the UID is stable, even though the posterior ligament complex, including the capsule of the involved joint, is disrupted and the posterior longitudinal ligament and annulus are partially disrupted. Braakman and Vinken (88) noted that the inferior facet of the dislocated joint is frequently fractured and that the capsule of the nondislocated (contralateral) interfacetal joint is also disrupted. Beatson (43) has demonstrated experimentally that it is impossible to produce forward displacement of the involved vertebra of more than one-half the width of a vertebral body in the presence of a UID.

> *The reader is reminded that "superior facet" refers to the superior facet of the apophyseal joint, i.e., the anatomic inferior facet of the upper vertebra.*

The concept of UID and the diagnostic radiographic significance of the rotational component of its mechanism of injury are clearly demonstrated by means of a dried, disarticulated cervical skeleton.

129

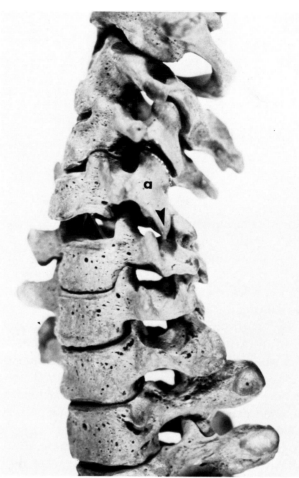

Figure 5.1. Oblique projection of a cervical skeleton showing a manipulated unilateral interfacetal dislocation of C_4 on C_5. The articular mass of C_4, including its inferior facet, is dislocated anterior to the subjacent articular mass of C_5. The posteroinferior aspect of the articular mass (*arrowhead*) is seated in the intervertebral foramen.

Figure 5.2 is the neutral lateral radiograph of such a specimen in which the contiguous articulating surfaces of one of the facetal joints at the C_3–C_4 level have been identified by lead foil. It is an important observation that the joint spaces and the posterior cortical surfaces of the articulating pillars at each level are superimposed upon one another in a true lateral projection.

Following dislocation of the marked joint, lateral and oblique radiographs were made of the specimen. The lateral radiograph (Fig. 5.3) demonstrates that the superior facet of the joint is dislocated anterior to its contiguous inferior facet. Below the level of dislocation, the vertebrae are seen in lateral position. At the level of dislocation and above, the vertebrae are seen in oblique position because of the rotational component of the mechanism of injury.

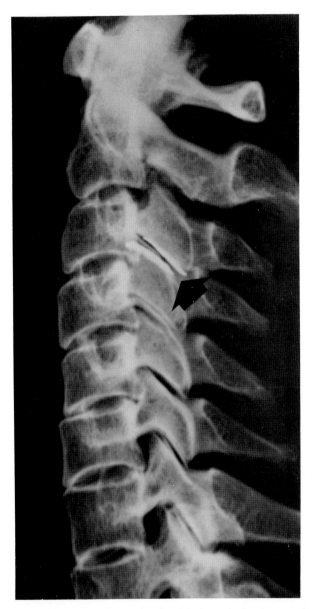

Figure 5.2. Neutral lateral radiograph of a dried cervical spine specimen in which the superior and inferior facets of one of the interfacetal joints at the C_3 on C_4 level have been marked with lead (*arrow*). The interfacetal joints are superimposed and are situated, normally, posterior to the vertebral body.

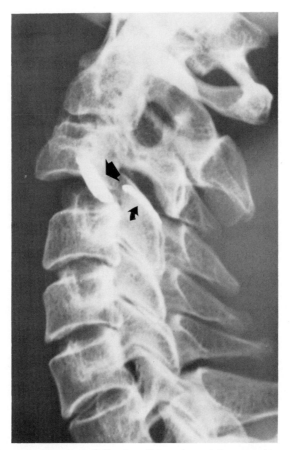

Figure 5.3.   Lateral radiograph following dislocation of the marked facetal joint. The dislocated superior facet (arrow) of the involved joint is clearly anterior to the contiguous inferior facet (*curved arrow*). At the level of dislocation and above, the vertebrae are seen in obliquity. Below the level of the dislocation, the vertebrae are seen in lateral position.

In the oblique radiograph of the same specimen (Fig. 5.4), the dislocated superior facet of the involved joint is clearly evident in the intervertebral foramen anterior to the inferior facet and its articular mass. Due to the effect of rotation, the second and third vertebrae are seen in nearly true lateral projection in this *oblique* view.

To illustrate the effect of rotation further, a UID was produced on the same side as the marked joint, but at the next subjacent level, and radiographs were again obtained in lateral and oblique projections.

In the lateral radiograph (Fig. 5.5), the marked facetal joint has been rotated anteriorly, along with all of the vertebrae above the level of dislocation, and is superimposed upon the vertebral bodies. Below the level of dislocation, the vertebrae are seen in lateral position, while those above the level of dislocation are recorded in nearly oblique view.

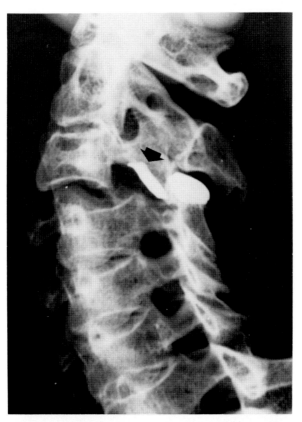

Figure 5.4. Oblique radiograph of same specimen as shown in Figure 5.3. The dislocated superior facet of the involved joint (*arrow*) lies in the intervertebral foramen. Below the level of the dislocation, the vertebrae are seen in oblique projection. At the level of dislocation and above, the vertebrae are nearly lateral in position.

In the oblique projection of this specimen (Fig. 5.6), the vertebrae above the level of the dislocation are seen in lateral projection because of the rotation inherent in the mechanism of injury of UID.

Radiographically, in the neutral lateral projection, the body of the dislocated vertebra of UID is typically anteriorly displaced a distance less than one-half the anteroposterior diameter of the vertebral body (Fig. 5.7) but more than the 1- to 3-mm forward translation frequently seen with anterior subluxation or hyperextension fracture-dislocation. The rotational component of the mechanism of injury is indicated by lack of superimposition of the articular masses and the interfacetal joints at the level of the dislocation and above. The dislocated articular mass, being rotated anteriorly, is partially superimposed upon and obscured by the vertebral body. All of the vertebrae above the level of dislocation are similarly rotated and present an identical roentgen appearance. The posterior inferior margin of the dislocated superior facet is seen in the intervertebral foramen anterior to the superior tip

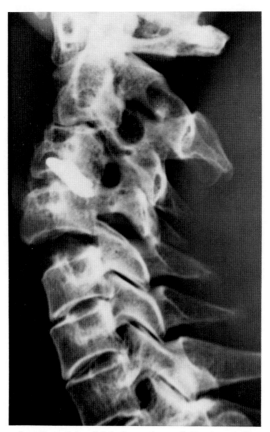

Figure 5.5. Lateral radiograph of dried specimen following unilateral dislocation on the same side as the marked facetal joint, but at the next lower level. Below the dislocation, the vertebrae are seen in lateral projection. Above the dislocation, the rotational component is indicated by the anterior location of the marked facetal joint and by the fact that the upper vertebrae are seen in oblique projection.

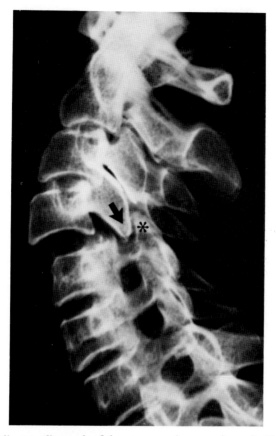

Figure 5.6.   Oblique radiograph of the same specimen as shown in Figure 5.5. Below the level of dislocation, the vertebrae are in oblique position. The relationship of the dislocated articular mass (*arrow*) to the subjacent mass (*) is clear. Above the level of dislocation, because of the rotational component, the vertebrae are seen in true lateral projection.

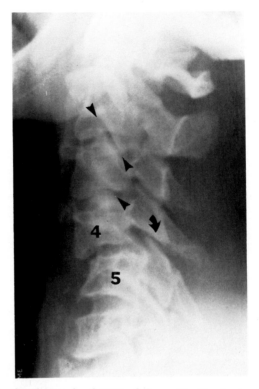

Figure 5.7. Lateral radiograph of UID of C_4 on C_5. The body of C_4 is anteriorly translated less than 50% of its anteroposterior diameter. The rotational component of UID is demonstrated by superimposition of the interfacetal joints on the side of dislocation being superimposed upon the vertebral bodies (*arrowheads*) above the level of dislocation, subluxation of the contralateral interfacetal joints at the level of dislocation (*curved arrow*), and only a single articular mass posterior to the vertebral bodies at the level of dislocation and above.

of the contiguous inferior facet and its articular mass (Fig. 5.8). As a result of the dislocation, the contiguous facets are no longer in apposition and are uncovered, or exposed. Hence, the term "naked" facet. Either of the articular masses of the involved joint may be fractured (Figs. 5.9 and 5.10) during dislocation. Tiny fragments from the margins of the facets are usually of no clinical significance. Large or comminuted fractures of the involved articular masses may render the UID unstable.

Increased interspinous and interlaminar distance ("fanning") (Fig. 5.10*a*) indicates disruption of the posterior ligament complex.

Oblique projections of the cervical spine are optimally obtained by positioning the patient, either erect or recumbent, so that the cervical spine is approximately 45° off the anteroposterior (coronal plane) position in each direction. (As previously discussed and illustrated (Fig. 1.44), oblique projections of diagnostic quality may be routinely obtained with the patient supine when the patient's condition precludes movement.) In the oblique projection of the dislocated side,

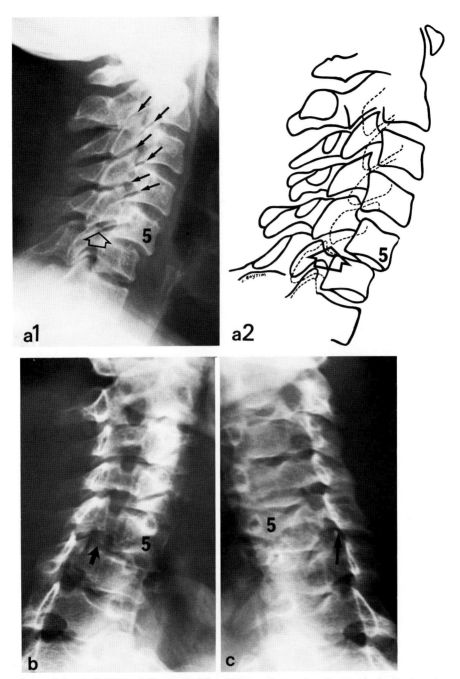

Figure 5.8. (*a1*) UID of C_5 on C_6. The dislocated vertebra is anteriorly displaced a distance less than one-half the anteroposterior diameter of the vertebral body. The posterior inferior corner of the dislocated superior facet (*open arrow*) is visible anterior to its contiguous inferior facet, seated in the intervertebral foramen. Above the level of dislocation, all of the facetal joints on the side of the dislocation, because of the rotational component of the injury, lie anterior to the contralateral facetal joint. Each set of *arrows* indicates the location of the facetal joints at the same level. In the schematic representation (*a2*), the facetal joints on the side of the dislocation are indicated by the *broken line*. (*b*) In the left posterior oblique projection, the dislocated superior facet (*arrow*) is seen in the intervertebral foramen. (*c*) In the right posterior oblique projection, the contralateral, nondisplaced lamina (*arrow*) is situated slightly superiorly and anteriorly with respect to the subjacent lamina, but it remains posterior to the subjacent lamina.

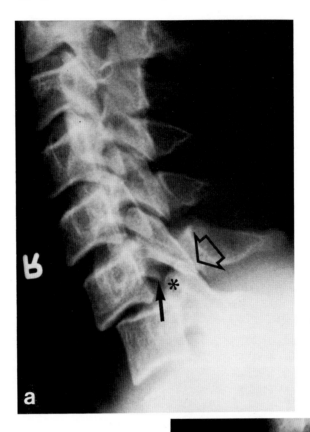

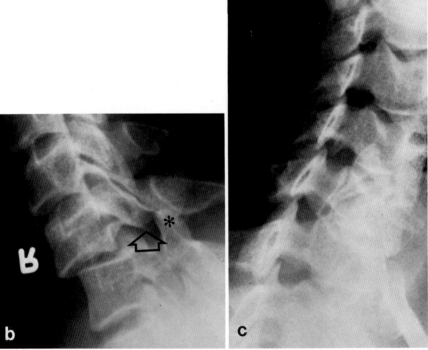

Figure 5.9.

UID is manifested by the dislocated articular mass seated in the inferior portion of the intervertebral foramen anterior to the subjacent articular mass (Figs. 5.9*b* and 5.10*b*). In oblique projections in which the articular masses are not well seen but the laminae are seen "end-on", UID is manifested by the lamina of the dislocated vertebra lying anterior to the subjacent lamina, thereby disrupting the normal "shingles-on-a-roof" alignment of the laminae (Figs. 5.11 and 5.12).

The oblique projection of the side opposite that of the dislocation demonstrates varying degrees of partial dislocation (subluxation) of the contralateral interfacetal joint (Fig. 5.10*c*). Maximum subluxation occurs when the contralateral articular mass (Fig. 5.8*c*) or lamina (Figs. 5.9*c* and 5.12*c*) comes to rest atop its subjacent counterpart. This relationship is referred to as the subluxed mass being "perched" upon the subjacent mass.

In the anteroposterior radiograph, UID is evidenced by rotation of the spinous processes from the level of the dislocation upward off the midline in the direction of the side of the dislocated interfacetal joint. Thus, the displaced spinous processes point to the side of the dislocation. The most caudad spinous process deviated from the midline indicates the level of dislocation (Fig. 5.13).

Although multiplanar CT usually provides little additional information to that obtained from the plain-film evaluation of UID and is therefore not routinely indicated in this injury, CT does identify related injuries of the involved vertebrae that may not be discernible on routine projections. Interfacetal dislocation is frequently difficult to identify on axial CT images because of the orientation of the plane of the CT beam to that of the articular masses and their interfacetal joints. Additionally, the average interfacetal vertical height of an adult articular mass is approximately 5 mm. CT "slices" greater than 5 mm thick may not record a UID. Consequently, axial CT images of 1-to 3-mm thickness are required to evaluate the posterior elements in the cervical spine adequately. Figure 5.14 compares the axial display of normal interfacetal joints and a UID. Figure 5.15 compares plain radiographs, multiplanar CT, and three-dimensional CT reformatted images of a patient with UID and associated fracture of the subjacent articular mass. The information provided by the sagittal and coronal

Figure 5.9. Unilateral interfacetal dislocation with a fracture of the dislocated superior facet. (*a*) Neutral lateral radiograph. The amputated, dislocated superior facet (small arrow) lies anterior to its contiguous inferior facet (∗). The contralateral superior facet (*open arrow*) has glided upward with respect to its contiguous inferior facet but retains its normal position posterior to the inferior facet. (*b*) In the right posterior oblique projection, the fractured, dislocated superior facet (*open arrow*) is clearly seen in the intervertebral foramen anterior to its contiguous inferior facet (∗). (*c*) In the opposite oblique projection, the alignment of the laminae is normal.

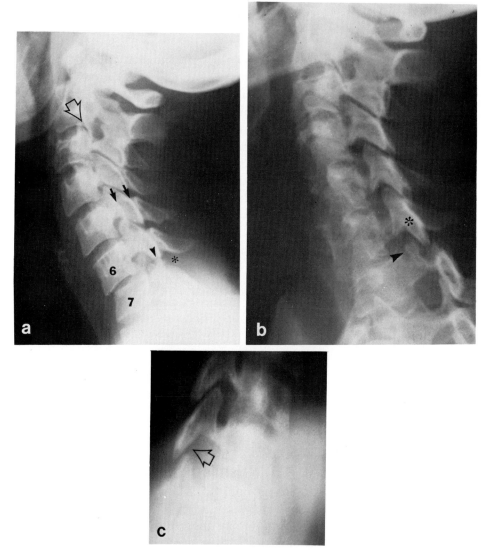

Figure 5.10. UID of C_6 on C_7. The neutral lateral projection (*a*) displays < 50% anterior translation of the C_6 body, subluxation of the contralateral interfacetal joint (*arrowhead*) and "fanning" (∗), all indicative of hyperflexion as well as lack of super-imposition of the posterior cortical margins of the articular masses (*double arrows*) and superimposition of the interfacetal joints upon the vertebral bodies (*open arrow*), indic-ative of rotation. In the oblique projection (*b*), the dislocated articular mass (∗) is seen seated in the inferior portion of the subjacent intervertebral foramen. The superior portion of the subjacent articular mass has been fractured and the separate fragment (*arrowhead*) has been displaced anteriorly, together with the dislocated articular mass, into the intervertebral foramen. Although this is an oblique projection, at the level of dislocation and above, the vertebrae are in more of a lateral than an oblique projec-tion, reflective of the rotational component of UID. On the opposite side (*c*) the con-tralateral facetal joint (*open arrow*) is subluxated.

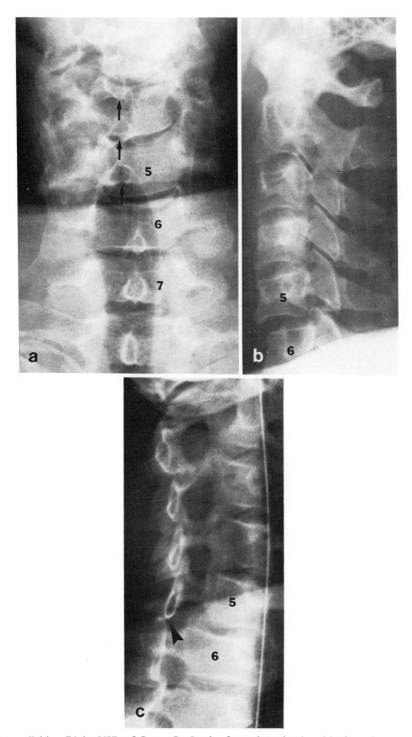

Figure 5.11. Right UID of C_5 on C_6. In the frontal projection (*a*), the spinous processes from C_5 (*arrows*) upward are deviated to the right while those of C_6, C_7, and T_1 remain midline. All of the radiographic signs of UID previously described in lateral projection are seen in part *b*. (From Grainger, R.C. and Allison, D.J.: *A Textbook of Organ Imaging*. New York, Churchill Livingstone, 1986, Chapter 68.) In the oblique projection (*c*), the normal shingling effect of the laminae seen end-on is disrupted in that the right lamina of C_5 (*arrowhead*) is situated anterior to that of C_6, indicating the site of UID.

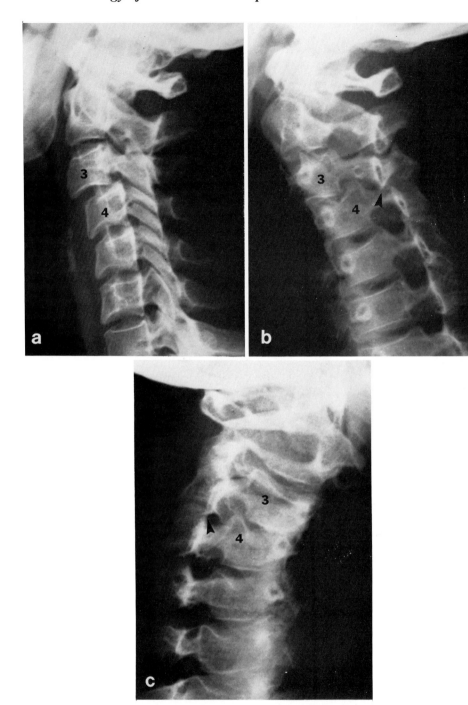

Figure 5.12.   Left UID of C_3 on C_4. In lateral projection (*a*), C_3 is anteriorly displaced a distance < 50% of the anteroposterior diameter of its body. In the left anterior oblique projection (*b*), the UID is indicated by the left lamina of C_2 lying anterior to that of C_3 (disruption of normal shingling) (*arrowhead*). In the opposite oblique (*c*), the contralateral lamina of C_2 is "perched" (*arrowhead*) upon that of C_3, indicating sub-luxation of this interfacetal joint.

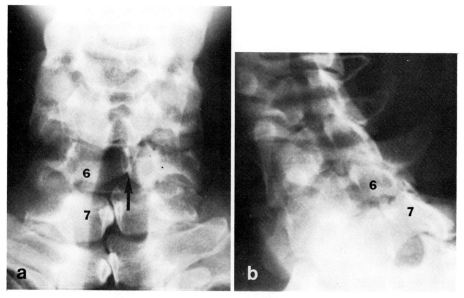

Figure 5.13. (*a*) Displacement of the spinous processes from the midline (*arrow*) toward the side of unilateral interfacetal dislocation. Bifid spinous processes of C_7 and T_1 are an incidental finding. The left anterior oblique projection (*b*) demonstrates the dislocated left articular mass of C_6 lying anterior to the articular mass of C_7.

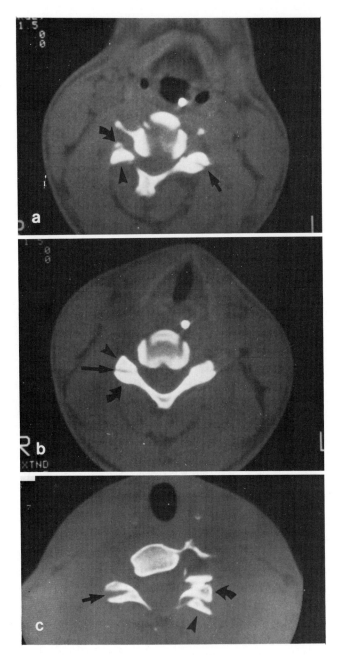

Figure 5.14. (*a*) Axial CT appearance of UID. The right interfacetal joint is dislocated with the tip of the dislocated supra-adjacent articular mass (*curved arrow*) seen in the intervertebral foramen anterior to its contiguous subjacent articular mass. As a result of the dislocation, the superior facet of the subjacent articular mass (*arrowhead*) is uncovered, producing the "exposed" or "naked" facet sign. Subluxation of the contralateral interfacetal joint is indicated by the asymmetry of its facets (*arrow*).

(*b*) The axial CT appearance of normal interfacetal joints at a different level in the same patient is shown for comparison. The articular masses of the vertebra above (*curved arrow*) are normally posterior to those of the subjacent vertebra (*arrowhead*). The lucency between (*arrow*) is the interfacetal joint space.

Part (*c*) is the axial CT scan of a second patient with UID on the left. This dislocated articular mass (*curved arrow*) lies anterior to its subjacent counterpart, the superior facet of which (*arrowhead*) is uncovered ("naked"). The contralateral interfacetal joint is subluxated (*arrow*).

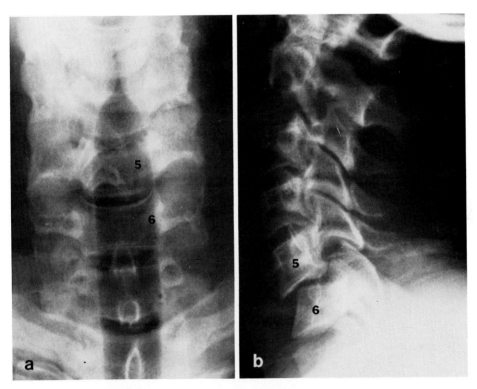

Figure 5.15.   Right UID of C_5 on C_6 in frontal (*a*), lateral (*b*), and right anterior oblique (*c*) projections. Axial CT (*d*) of the same patient demonstrates the anterior dislocation of the right articular mass of C_5 (*arrowhead*) with respect to the subjacent articular mass of C_6 and the "naked" superior facet of C_6 (*arrow*). Reformatted sagittal projections of the right lateral column (*e*) demonstrate the interfacetal joint dislocation (*arrow*) and sagittal reformation at a comparable level on the left (*f*) demonstrates a subluxated ("perched") contralateral interfacetal joint (*arrow*). A fracture of the right superior facet of C_6, unrecognized on plain films or conventional CT, is clearly evident on the 3-D reformatted images (*g* and *h*, *arrows*). (*i*) The inferior facet (*arrows*) of the dislocated right articular mass of C_5 is clearly evident in the intervertebral foramen on the 3-D reformatted image seen from below upward. *j* and *k* are reformations with the spine sectioned in the midsagittal plane and the left half removed so that the right half of the spinal canal is seen from within. In the lateral projection (*j*) and the one seen from below upward (*k*), the right lamina of dislocated C_5 is clearly seen to lie medial to the right lamina of C_6. This is the pathologic basis of disruption of the normal laminar "shingling" that is characteristic of UID on the oblique plain radiograph.

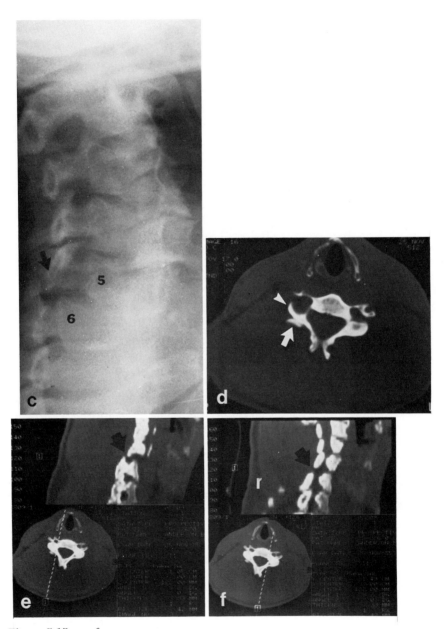

Figure 5.15.   *c–f.*

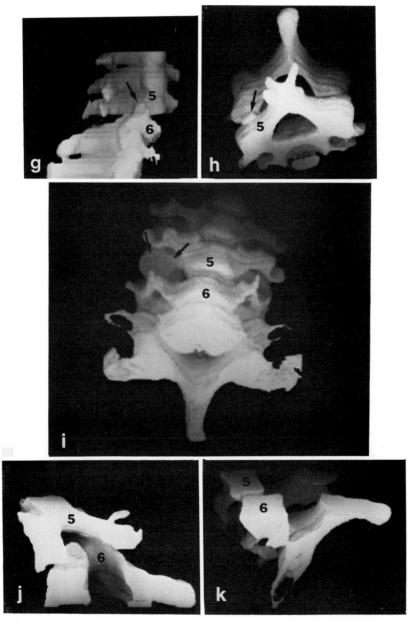

Figure 5.15. *g–k.*

images is only grossly useful because they are degraded by the reformation process even when high-resolution techniques are employed. Three-dimensional reformation greatly facilitates conceptualization of UID by presenting a visually integrated image of the spine as opposed to the multiplanar data that must be mentally integrated into a composite image. In addition, three-dimensional CT frequently demonstrates clinically significant injuries not appreciated on plain-film or multiplanar CT studies (33).

Chapter 6

Simultaneous Hyperextension and Rotation: Pillar Fracture

The combination of hyperextension and rotation of the cervical spine has also been called "unilateral extension" by Whitley and Forsyth (52). With this mechanism of injury, the maximum force is concentrated on the "lateral column," resulting in fracture of an articular mass ("pillar") on the side in the direction of the rotation. The pillar fracture is not a common injury, but Smith (94) believes it may occur more commonly than has been reported.

Pathologically, the causative force results in a fracture that principally involves the articular mass as the mass is compressed between its contiguous superior and subjacent counterparts. Infrequently, adjacent masses may be fractured.

The pillar fracture is usually vertical or obliquely vertical and is usually simple or only minimally comminuted, suggesting that the involved mass was split from above downward by the impact of the posterior marginal cortex of the inferior facet of the superior vertebra. In this variety of pillar fracture, the separate fragment is usually posteriorly or posterolaterally displaced. Infrequently, the articular mass may be severely comminuted, giving the impression of having been crushed between the adjacent masses. The mass fracture may extend anteriorly to involve the transverse process, the pedicle, or both, or posteriorly into the lamina. The interfacetal joint above the involved mass is frequently disrupted.

Radiographically, the pillar fracture may be easily overlooked on routine frontal and lateral projections. However, frequently subtle changes occur on the frontal and lateral radiographs that should create a high index of suspicion regarding the presence of a pillar fracture. Oblique and/or pillar views usually demonstrate the pillar fracture very clearly.

In the anteroposterior radiograph, displacment of the pillar fragments disrupts the smoothly undulating, seemingly continuous cortical

149

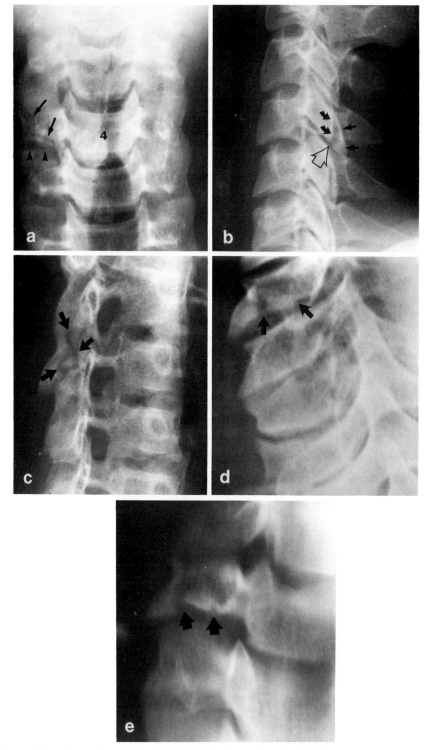

Figure 6.1 Right pillar fracture of C$_4$. In the frontal projection (*a*), the lateral margin of the lateral mass is disrupted, the articular mass fracture is indicated by the *arrows*, and the interfacetal joint space is indicated by the *arrowheads*. In the lateral projection (*b*) the "double outline" sign is formed by the posterior cortex of the displaced fragment of the right articular mass fracture (*arrow*) and the posterior cortex of the intact contralateral mass (*curved arrows*). A fracture of the inferior facet of the right articular mass is indicated by the *open arrow*. The articular mass fracture (*arrows*) is clearly delineated in the right anterior oblique projection (*c*), the pillar view (*d*) and the tomogram obtained in the pillar view position (*e*).

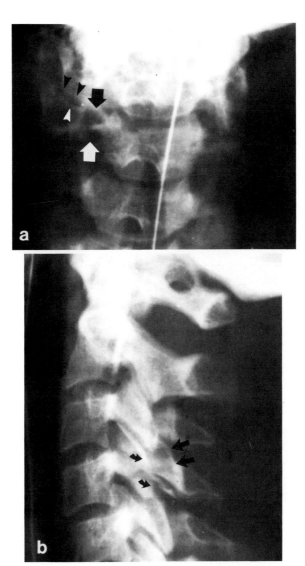

Figure 6.2. Pillar fracture of the right articular mass of C_4. In the frontal projection (*a*), a vertical fracture line (*arrows*) separates the articular mass from the body of C_4. The lateral mass is laterally displaced, resulting in disruption of the lateral margin of the "lateral column" and causing interfacetal joints (*arrowheads*) to become visible. In the lateral radiograph (*b*), the posterior fragment of the mass fracture is posteriorly displaced and the relationship of its posterior cortex (*arrows*) to that of the contralateral mass (*curved arrows*) results in the "double outline" sign. The comminuted lateral mass (pillar) fracture is clearly seen in the right anterior oblique projection (*c*). (The left anterior oblique projection (*d*) is shown for comparison.) The axial CT (*e*) demonstrates comminution of the right articular mass and the extent of the fracture into the transverse process (*arrowheads*) confinement of the fracture (*arrows*) to the lateral column without encroachment of the spinal canal is clearly demonstrated in the coronally reformatted image of the metrizamide CT myelogram (*f*).

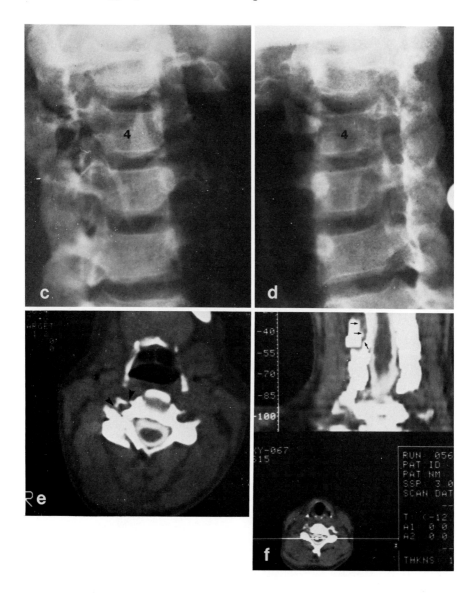

margin of the "lateral column" at the level of the mass ("pillar") fractures (Figs. 6.1 and 6.2) or disrupt the lateral column itself (Figs. 6.3 and 6.4). The interfacetal joint spaces, not normally visible on the frontal projection, may be partially evident at the level of the fracture due to rotation of the fragment(s) (Figs. 6.1, 6.2, and 6.4) (94). In the lateral projection, localized lack of superimposition of the posterior cortical margins of the articular masses at the same level (the "double outline" sign (94)) (Figs. 6.1*b*, 6.3*b*, and 6.5) is the result of posterior displacement of the separate mass fragment. A fracture line or defect may be visible in the inferior articulating facet of the involved mass (Fig. 6.1*b*).

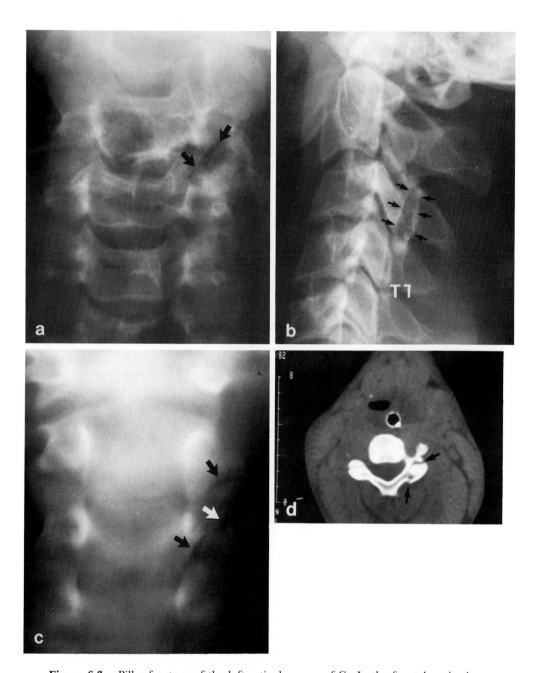

Figure 6.3. Pillar fracture of the left articular mass of C_3. In the frontal projection (*a*), an obvious comminuted fracture (*arrows*) is present in the "lateral column" at the level of C_3. The "double outline" sign (*arrows*) involving C_3 is seen in the lateral projection (*b*). Comminution of the fracture (*arrows*) is confirmed in the frontal polydirectional tomogram (*c*), and limitation of the fracture to the articular mass (*arrows*), is shown in the axial CT scan (*d*). In this patient, the fracture was limited to the articular mass and did not extend into the transverse process.

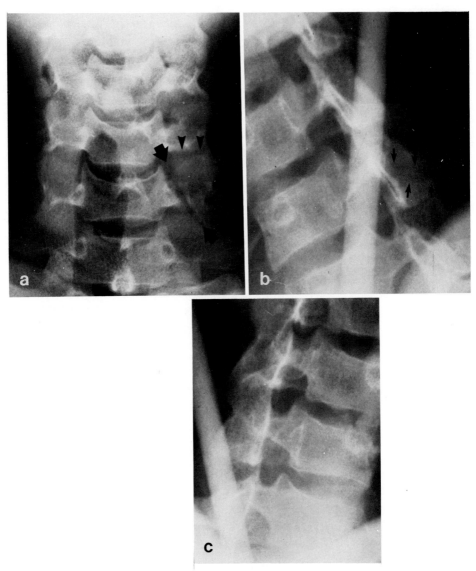

Figure 6.4.   Pillar fracture of C_6 on the left. In the frontal projection (*a*), the fracture (*arrows*) is clearly evident in the "lateral column." The C_5–C_6 interfacetal joint is visible as a transverse lucency (*arrowheads*). The fracture of the left articular mass (pillar) of C_6 (*arrows*) is evident in the left anterior oblique projection (*b*). The intact right articular mass of C_6 is seen in the right anterior oblique projection (*c*) (shown for comparison).

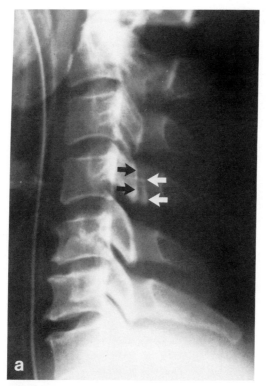

Figure 6.5.   Pillar fracture of the left articular mass of C_4. The "double outline" sign of C_4 (*arrows*) is seen in the lateral projection (*a*). Fracture lines and disruption of the lateral margin of the "lateral column" (*arrows*) are present in the anteroposterior radiograph (b) and are seen to better advantage in the frontal polydirectional tomogram (*arrows*) (*c*). The comminuted fracture of the articular mass is particularly well demonstrated in the lateral polydirectional tomogram (*d*) as is subluxation of the C_4–C_5 interfacetal joint. Comminution of the articular mass fracture (*arrows*) with extension into the transverse process and impingement upon the foramen transversarium (*arrowhead*) is clearly seen in the axial CT images (*e* and *f*).

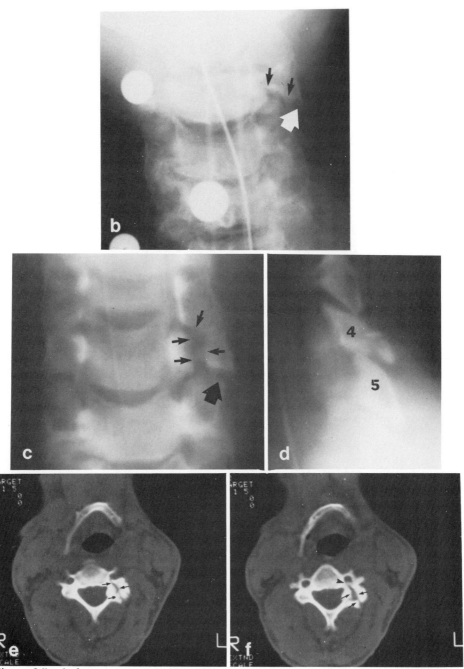

Figure 6.5.   *b–f.*

The pillar fracture is usually readily apparent on the appropriate oblique projections (Figs. 6.1*c*, 6.2*c*, and 6.4*b*). However, it may not be visible on oblique projections if the fragments are neither displaced nor depressed or if the vertical plane of the fracture line does not coincide with the obliquity of the projection.

The pillar view, because it is designed to depict the lateral masses *en face*, provides optimum plain-film visualization of an articular mass fracture. The fracture typically extends vertically through the articular mass, and the separate fragments may be depressed or posteriorly or laterally displaced (Figs. 6.1*b–e*). Rectilinear or polydirectional tomography enhances demonstration of the pillar fracture in frontal (Fig. 6.3*c*), lateral (Fig. 6.5*d*), oblique (Fig. 6.1*c*), or pillar (Fig. 6.1*d* and *e*) projections.

Axial computed tomography optimally demonstrates the extent of the pillar fracture and the integrity of the foramen transversarium and the spinal canal (Figs. 6.2, 6.3, and 6.5).

The diagnosis of an acute pillar fracture requires the demonstration of an acute fracture line or defect involving the articular mass. Asymmetry of lateral masses, on the same side or on opposite sides at the same level, is a common radiographic finding unrelated to patient age and of protein etiology, including developmental. Thus, variations from the normal configuration of the articular mass alone, without a demonstrable fracture line, should not be used as evidence of an acute pillar fracture (43,95).

Chapter 7

Vertical Compression Injuries

Most authorities recognize vertical compression injuries as a distinct type of cervical spine trauma (38,41,43,47,48,50,52,66,100–103). The principal dissent from this consensus is that of Selecki and Williams (51), who believe that compression is such a major factor in all types of cervical trauma that "any classification of mechanism of injury in which it is implied that there is a single mechanism for compression fractures is bound to confuse the mechanisms with the radiological end results of the injury."

Vertical compression injuries occur only in those segments of the spine that are capable of being voluntarily straightened, i.e., the cervical and lumbar regions (21,47). Cervical compression injuries are usually the result of force transmitted through the skull and occipital condyles to the spine at the precise instant that the spine is straight. The same type of force applied through the skull with the spine flexed or extended results in hyperflexion or hyperextension injuries.

Compression injuries of the cervical spine are (*a*) the Jefferson bursting fracture of the atlas and (*b*) the "burst" or "bursting" fracture of the lower cervical spine.

THE JEFFERSON FRACTURE OF THE ATLAS

The bursting fracture of the atlas was first described by Jefferson (97) in 1920. Until 1970 only 191 cases of this injury had been reported in the world literature (41). The fracture is the result of force transmitted from the vertex of the skull through the occipital condyles to the lateral masses of the atlas, driving each laterally.

Jefferson's original description (97) was that of a *bilateral* fracture of both the anterior and the posterior arches of C_1 (Fig. 7.1). Pathologically, the Jefferson bursting fracture consists simply of disruption of both the anterior and posterior arches of C_1. Computed tomography has demonstrated that the arch fractures may be unilateral (Fig. 7.2) as well as bilateral. The transverse atlantal ligament may remain intact or be partially or completely disrupted. Disruption of the trans-

158

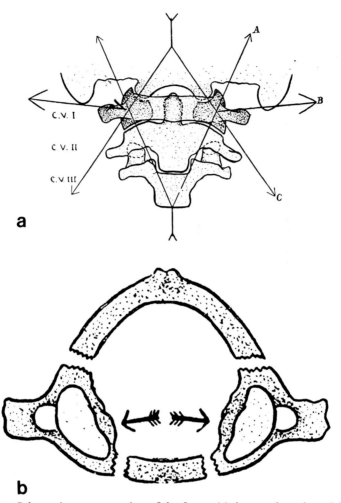

a

b

Figure 7.1.   Schematic representation of the forces (*a*) that produce the axial loading fracture of the atlas and of the fracture (*b*) itself as originally described by Jefferson. Note that Jefferson's original description consisted of bilateral fractures of both the anterior and the posterior arches. (From Jefferson, G.: Fracture of the atlas vertebra. Report of four cases, and a review of those previously recorded. *Br. J. Surg.* 7:407, 1920.)

verse atlantal ligament may result in widening of the anterior or lateral atlantodental intervals.

Isolated rupture of the transverse atlantal ligament is a rare injury (141) that, by definition, occurs without associated atlas or axis fracture. In spite of the absence of an atlas or axis fracture, disruption of the transverse atlantal ligament results in atlantoaxial instability. On lateral plain radiography and axial CT, isolated rupture of the transverse atlantal ligament is demonstrated by an increase in the width of the anterior atlantodental interval (AADI) and the absence of associated fracture (Fig. 7.3).

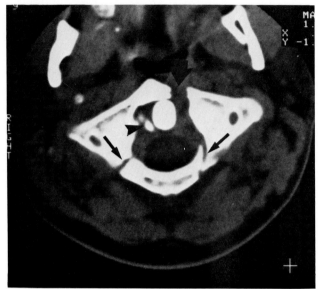

Figure 7.2. Jefferson bursting fracture with only a single fracture of the anterior arch and bilateral fracture of the posterior arch (*arrows*). A small fragment (*arrowhead*) has been avulsed from the medial surface of the right articular mass of C_1 by the intact transverse atlantal ligament.

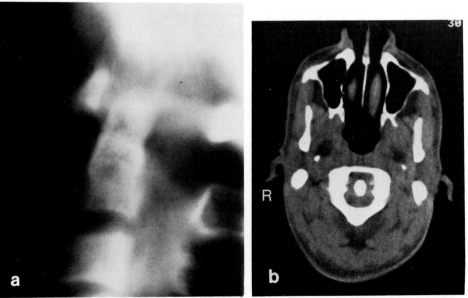

Figure 7.3. Isolated rupture of the transverse atlantal ligament is indicated on plain (*a*) and axial computed (*b*) tomograms by the increase in width of the anterior atlantodental interval and the absence of associated atlantal or axial fracture.

The Jefferson bursting fracture may be associated with a vertical fracture through one, or both, of the articular masses where the larger separate lateral fragment is laterally displaced while the smaller medial fragment maintains a normal relationship to the dens by virtue of the intact transverse atlantal ligament (Fig. 7.4). The significance of this

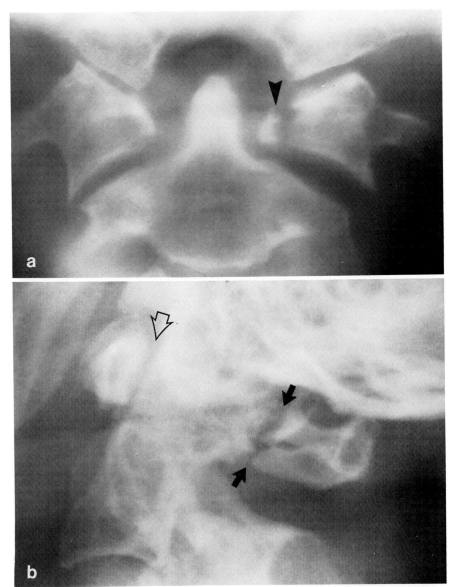

Figure 7.4. Polydirectional tomogram (*a*) of a Jefferson bursting fracture with an avulsion fracture of the medial surface of the left articular mass (*arrowhead*) indicative of an intact transverse atlantal ligament. In the lateral radiograph (*b*), the normal anterior atlantodental interval (*open arrow*) confirms the intact transverse atlantal ligament, and the posterior arch fractures (*arrows*) complete the radiographic signs of a Jefferson bursting fracture.

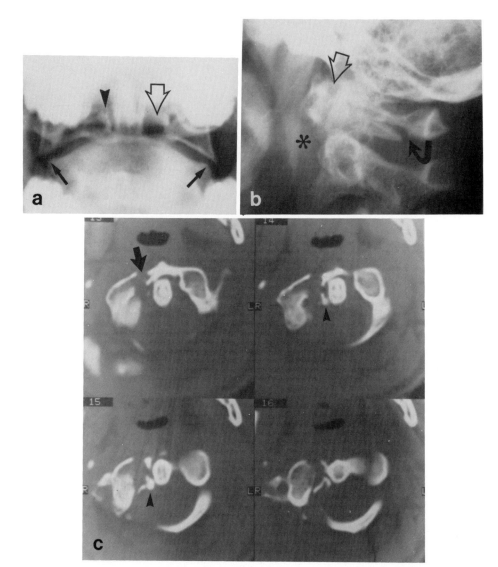

Figure 7.5. Jefferson bursting fracture with avulsion fracture of the right articular mass and intact transverse atlantal ligament. In the open-mouth projection (*a*), the Jefferson bursting fracture is indicated by the bilateral lateral displacement of the lateral masses, asymmetry of the lateral margins of the articulating facets of C_1–C_2 (*arrows*), and abnormal width of the left lateral atlantodental interval (*open arrow*). The thin, vertical avulsion fracture of the medial surface of the right articular mass of C_1 (*arrowhead*), indicates an intact transverse atlantal ligament. In the lateral projection (*b*), the normal anterior atlantodental interval (*open arrow*) confirms the intact transverse atlantal ligament. The cervicocranial prevertebral soft tissue swelling (*) reflects the hematoma secondary to the anterior arch fracture. The posterior arch fracture is indicated by the *curved arrow*. Axial CT (*c*), establishes the right (unilateral) anterior arch fracture (*arrow*) and confirms the avulsion fracture of the right articular mass (*arrowhead*). The posterior arch fractures were not demonstrated on these axial scans.

variant of the Jefferson fracture is that while lateral displacement of an intact articular mass of the atlas may be indicative of transverse atlantal ligament disruption, lateral displacement of only the lateral fragment of an atlas articular mass fracture is consistent with an intact transverse atlantal ligament. The former circumstance usually implies atlantoaxial instability, whereas the latter is consistent with atlantoaxial stability.

Radiographically, in the "open-mouth" projection of the atlantoaxial articulation, the classic Jefferson bursting fracture is characterized by essentially symmetrical bilateral lateral displacement of the articular masses of the atlas (Fig. 7.5). In the lateral projection, the diagnosis of a minimally displaced Jefferson bursting fracture or one associated with an intact transverse atlantal ligament can only be inferred on the basis of the posterior arch fracture and cervicocranial prevertebral soft tissue swelling because the anterior arch fractures are not visible in this projection (Fig. 7.6). The cervicocranial prever-

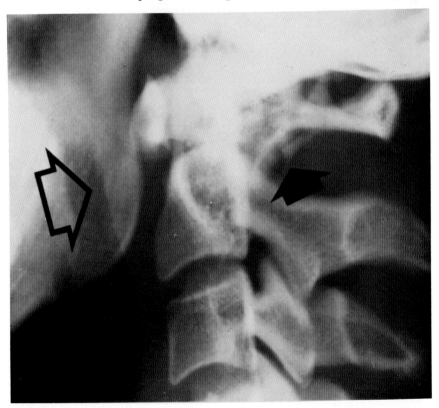

Figure 7.6. Jefferson fracture with minimal displacement of the posterior arch fragments (*solid arrow*). The most striking roentgen sign of the fracture is the abnormal thickness of the prevertebral soft tissues in the cervicocranium (*open arrow*), representing edema and hemorrhage secondary to the anterior arch component of this injury. (From Harris, J.H., Jr. and Harris, W.H.: *The Radiology of Emergency Medicine.* Baltimore, Williams & Wilkins, 1981.)

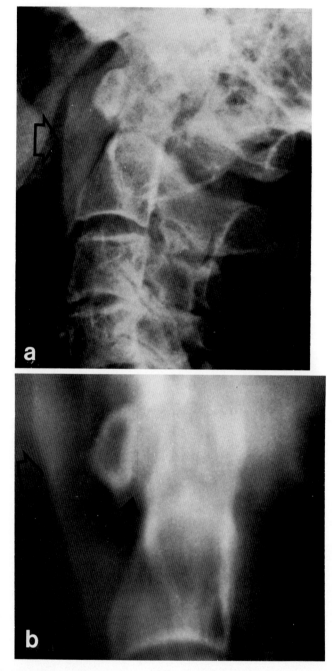

Figure 7.7. Cervicocranial soft tissue swelling (*open arrow*) is the most striking radiographic finding on the lateral radiograph (*a*) of this patient with a Jefferson bursting fracture. The lateral tomogram (*b*) confirms the presence of a cervicocranial hematoma and, in addition, demonstrates abnormal widening of the anterior atlantodental interval (*arrow*), consistent with at least partial disruption of the transverse atlantal ligament.

tebral soft tissue swelling may be the most prominent sign of a subtle Jefferson bursting fracture on lateral projection (Fig. 7.7*a*).

Anteroposterior plain-film or computed tomography is frequently required to establish the bilateral lateral mass displacement (Fig. 7.8), the extent and location of the atlas fractures, and, as previously indicated, the width of the atlantodental interval (Fig. 7.7*b*).

If the causative force of a Jefferson bursting fracture is eccentrically delivered to the vertex of the skull, the lateral displacement of articular masses may be dissimilar or asymmetrical (Fig. 7.9).

The Jefferson bursting fracture is clearly demonstrated by axial CT (Figs. 7.2 and 7.5) or by plain-film tomography (Figs. 7.4, 7.8, and 7.9).

Partial disruption of the transverse atlantal ligament, associated with Jefferson bursting fracture, is indicated by an increase in the AADI to between 3–5 mm, while an AADI in excess of 6 mm indicates complete disruption of the transverse atlantal ligament (141), unless this interval is widened by erosion of the dens and/or attenuation of the transverse atlantal ligament such as may occur in rheumatoid arthritis or Down's syndrome.

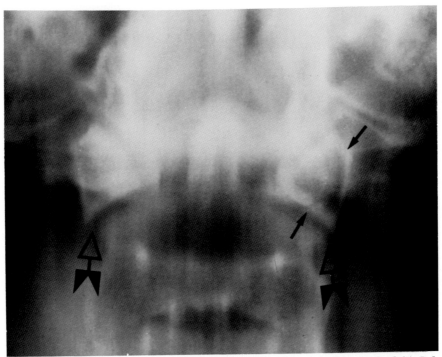

Figure 7.8. The lateral displacement of the lateral masses (*winged arrows*) of this Jefferson fracture was not apparent on the plain open-mouth view. The *small arrows* indicate a fracture of the left lateral mass of the atlas that, also was not visible on the routine radiograph. (From Harris, J.H., Jr. and Harris, W.H.: *The Radiology of Emergency Medicine*, ed 2. Baltimore, Williams & Wilkins, 1981.)

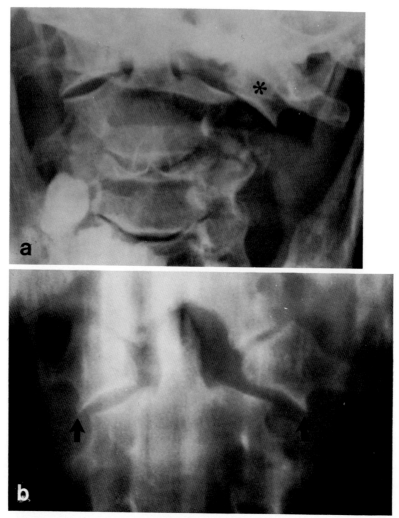

Figure 7.9.   This patient sustained a Jefferson bursting fracture as a result of a blow delivered to the right side of the vertex of the skull. In the "open-mouth" (*a*) radiograph, the severely laterally displaced left lateral mass of C_1 (∗) is clearly evident, as is the severely comminuted fracture of the left lateral aspect of the bodies of C_2 and C_3. The plain-film tomogram (*b*) confirms that each articular mass of the atlas is laterally displaced (*arrows*).

Conditions that might be mistaken for a Jefferson bursting fracture in the lateral projection include the isolated fracture of the posterior arch of the atlas and congenital failure of fusion of the posterior arch of C_1. The isolated fracture of the posterior arch of C_1 is one of the hyperextension family of cervical spine injuries. The absence of cervicocranial prevertebral soft tissue swelling (Fig. 7.10) distinguishes the isolated posterior arch fracture from the Jefferson bursting fracture on the lateral radiograph. However, the distinction can only be

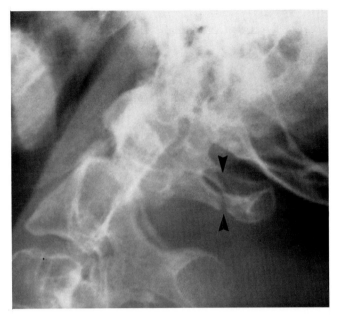

Figure 7.10. Isolated fracture of the posterior arch of the atlas (*arrowheads*). Absence of cervicocranial prevertebral soft tissue swelling is good presumptive evidence that the anterior arch of the atlas is intact.

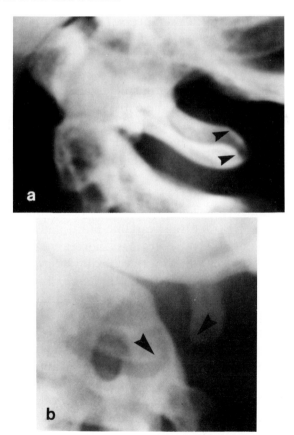

Figure 7.11. Congenital failure of fusion of the posterior arch of C_1 in lateral (*a*) and oblique (*b*) projections. The smoothly corticated margins of the unfused laminae (*arrowheads*) distinguish this anomaly from the isolated fracture of the posterior arch of C_1.

confirmed by demonstrating an intact anterior arch of C_1 by CT. The unfused posterior arch of C_1 is a congenital anomaly that is characterized by a smoothly corticated defect in the posterior aspect of the posterior arch, the absence of a posterior laminal line, and normal cervicocranial prevertebral soft tissues (Fig. 7.11). This anomaly may be best demonstrated in oblique projections of the cervical spine.

"BURSTING" FRACTURE OF THE LOWER CERVICAL SPINE

The vertical compression injury occurring in the lower cervical spine is referred to as the "burst," "bursting," "dispersion," "compression," or "axial loading" fracture. Roaf (38,50,61,66,98) has observed experimentally that the axial loading force transmitted to the lower cervical spine is dissipated by compression of an intervertebral disk. At that level, the compression of the disk causes the annulus to bulge circumferentially. With the annulus intact, the increased pressure within the intervertebral disk causes the liquid nucleus pulposus to implode through the inferior end-plate of the supra-adjacent vertebral body. The resultant abrupt increase in pressure within the vertebral body causes the centrum to explode from within outward, resulting in comminution of the vertebral body with variable degrees of centrifugal displacement of the fragments. The posterior fragments, being retropulsed a variable distance into the spinal canal, may impinge on or penetrate the ventral surface of the cord. White and Panjabi (18) refer to this injury as the "vertical compression" fracture and describe its mechanism as "presumably due to vertical force vector which causes an explosive failure with a variable amount of cord compression."

Retropulsion of posterior body fragments is characteristic of the bursting fracture. When the fragment is small and thin, it may not be visible on plain films (43). The extent of the neurologic deficit associated with the bursting fracture is variable but usually of lesser magnitude than the instant permanent acute anterior column syndrome characteristically associated with the flexion teardrop fracture of Schneider (85). In the lateral radiograph, the bursting fracture of the lower cervical spine may resemble the flexion teardrop fracture. When associated with permanent quadriplegia, the bursting fracture may also clinically resemble the flexion teardrop fracture. For these reasons, a few authors (51,73,99) consider the bursting fracture to be simply a variant of the flexion teardrop fracture. The great majority of authors, however, consider the bursting fracture of the lower cervical spine caused by vertical compression (axial loading) vector force to be a distinct entity separate from the flexion teardrop fracture caused by hyperflexion.

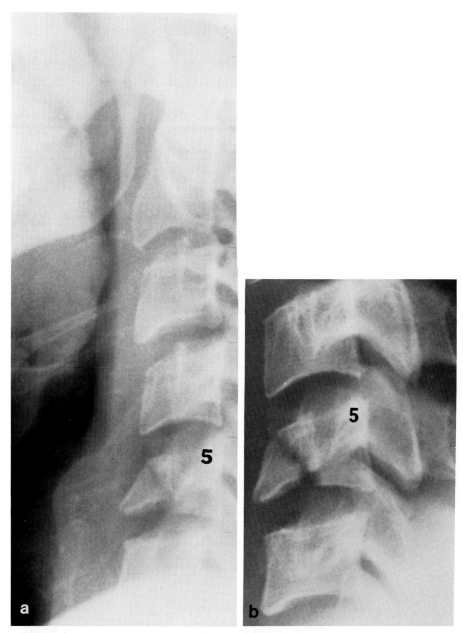

Figure 7.12. Bursting fracture of C_5. The lateral radiograph (*a*) demonstrates the straight attitude of the cervical segments, comminution of the body of C_5, and only minimal retropulsion of its posterior fragments. Comminution of the body of C_5 with loss of stature and minimal retropulsion of the posterior fragments is better demonstrated in the close-up view (*b*). In addition, the posterior column is intact and none of the signs of posterior column distraction, a feature of hyperflexion, is present.

The bursting fracture covers a wide spectrum of clinical and radiographic presentations. Clinically, the neurologic deficit ranges from transient paresthesia of the upper extremities to complete, permanent quadriplegia. Radiographically, in lateral projection, the appearance of the involved centrum may range from minimal comminution with minimal compression and displacement of fragments (Fig. 7.12) to severe comminution and compression with marked dispersion of fragments, particularly posteriorly (Fig. 7.13). The marked variation in clinical and radiographic findings of the bursting fracture differs dramatically from the single neurologic syndrome and typical radiographic appearance of the flexion teardrop fracture (Fig. 7.14). Appreciation of these differences has an important, practical clinical application relative to patient management. Because the neurologic deficit associated with the bursting fracture, including initial paraple-

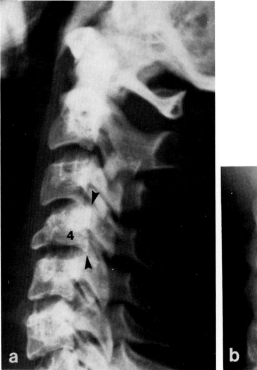
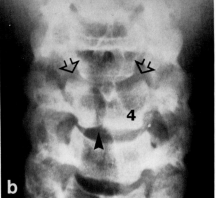

Figure 7.13. Lateral radiograph (*a*) of a bursting fracture of C$_4$ with severe comminution of the centrum and retropulsion of posterior fragments (*arrowheads*) into the spinal canal. Note the essentially normal attitude of the cervical spine and the absence of signs of posterior column distraction which distinguished this injury from the flexion teardrop fracture. The frontal projection (*b*) demonstrates the characteristic vertical fracture of the centrum (*arrowhead*). Dispersion of the fragments is evidenced by lateral displacement of the major fragments and disruption of the C$_5$–C$_6$ Luschka joints (*open arrows*).

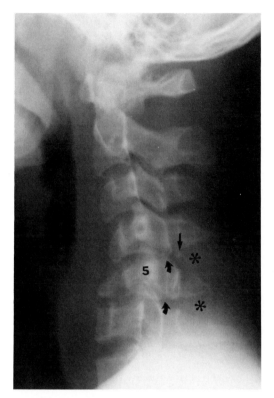

Figure 7.14. Flexion teardrop fracture of C_5. A severe hyperkyphosis exists at the C_5 level indicating a hyperflexion vector force. Consequently, the anterior column (vertebral body) is compressed resulting in anterior wedging, the large triangular fragment ("teardrop") and posterior angulation of the large body fragment as flexion occurred about the X axis. Inherent in hyperflexion is reciprocal distraction of the posterior column with widening of the interspinous and interlaminar spaces ("fanning") (∗) and subluxation of the interfacetal joints (*curved arrows*) at the C_4 and C_5 levels. A small fragment (*arrow*) has been avulsed from the superior margin of the lamina of C_5, which is also a hyperflexion phenomenon. Diffuse prevertebral soft tissue swelling indicates hemorrhage secondary to the anterior column musculoskeletal injury.

gia, may be transient, it is imperative that the radiographic characteristics of the bursting fracture be recognized so that the patient may be managed expectantly and the cervical cord especially protected.

Radiographically, in frontal projection the burst fracture is characterized by a vertical fracture line that extends through the height of the involved vertebral body (Figs. 7.12 and 7.13). This fracture defect, which is usually midline but may be eccentric (Fig. 7.15), distinguishes the bursting fracture from the wedge fracture which may resemble the bursting fracture in the lateral radiograph. In the frontal projection, the magnitude of dispersion is indicated by the amount of lateral displacement of the fragments and disruption of the Luschka joints (Figs. 7.13*b* and 7.16*b*).

In the lateral radiograph of the bursting fracture, the overall orientation of the cervical vertebrae is that of straightening or minor reversal of cervical lordosis (Figs. 7.12 and 7.13). Specifically, the cervical spine does not assume the flexed attitude characteristic of the flexion teardrop fracture. Therefore, the bursting fracture is characterized by the *absence* of signs of distraction of the posterior column of the spine, namely the absence of "fanning" and of bilateral interfacetal subluxation or dislocation, which are features of flexion. In the bursting fracture, the involved vertebral body is comminuted with the degree of comminution ranging from a few millimeters (Fig. 7.16) to severe comminution with many fragments (Fig. 7.17). Variable degrees of retropulsion of the posterior body fragments into the spinal canal are also characteristic of the bursting fracture (Figs. 7.12, 7.13, 7.17, and 7.18).

Traditional definitions of the bursting fracture describe a fracture limited to the vertebral body with intact posterior elements, including interfacetal joints and laminae (21,47,48,50,61,98,142). Axial computed tomography has demonstrated that while the articular masses and interfacetal joints are intact, the bursting fracture of the lower cervical spine typically includes a unilateral or bilateral laminar fracture as well (Figs. 7.17 and 7.19).

Plain-film recognition of a bursting fracture may be very difficult, if not impossible, when dispersion of the fragments and loss of vertebral body height are minimal (Fig. 7.19). A corollary of this observa-

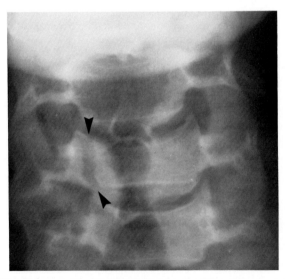

Figure 7.15. Atypical eccentric location (*arrowhead*) of the characteristic vertical vertebral body fracture of the bursting fracture of the lower cervical spine.

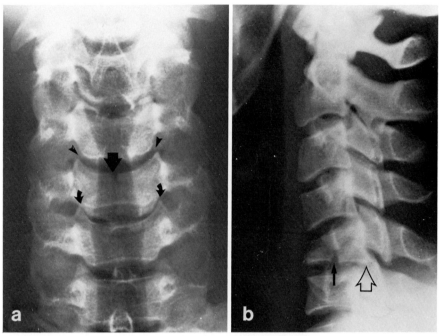

Figure 7.16. "Bursting" fracture of C₅ in frontal projection (*a*). The arrow indicates the vertical fracture of the vertebral body which is characteristic of this lesion. The C₄–C₅ Luschka joints are slightly widened (*arrowheads*) and the C₅–C₆ joints slightly narrowed (*curved arrow*), reflecting lateral dispersion of the major fragments. In the lateral projection (*b*), the cervical vertebrae are in vertical alignment. The body of C₅ is comminuted with a fracture defect of the inferior end-plate (*solid arrow*) and posterior displacement of the posterior body fragment (*open arrow*). The disk space is narrowed and the annulus bulges anteriorly. The interfacetal joints at the level of injury are neither subluxated nor dislocated and the interspinous ligament is intact, as evidenced by the absence of "fanning" of the interspinous space.

tion is that a small percentage of patients sustain simultaneous bursting fractures of adjacent vertebrae with only one of the fractures, usually the superiormost, being recognizable on the plain radiographs (Figs. 7.19 and 7.20). It is for these reasons that computed tomography should be mandatory for all patients in whom the radiographic findings do not match the clinical findings or in whom a bursting fracture is identified on plain films.

Recognition of the bursting fracture of the lower cervical spine is of great clinical importance because the distinction between it and the flexion teardrop fracture, particularly when associated with paraplegia, may only be established on the basis of the radiographic characteristics of the fracture. Because some divergence of opinion concerning the bursting fracture and the flexion teardrop fracture exists in the literature, several additional examples of bursting fractures are

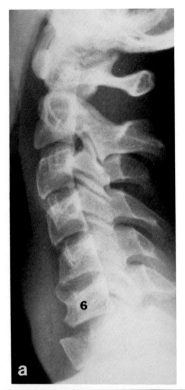

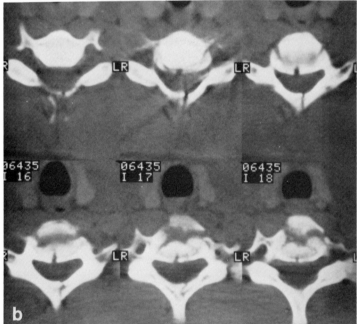

Figure 7.17. Severely comminuted bursting fracture of C₇ seen in lateral projection (*a*) and on axial CT (*b*). The extent of comminution and the degree of dispersion of the fragments, including retropulsion into the spinal canal, are thoroughly delineated on the axial images.

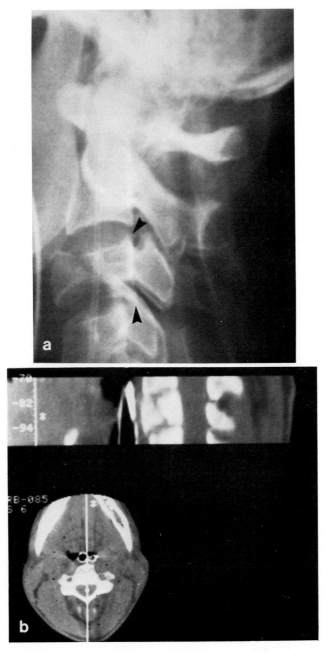

Figure 7.18.   Bursting fracture of C_3 in lateral projection (*a*) and sagittal reformation (*b*). While retropulsion of the posterior fragment (*arrowheads*) is evident in the plain radiograph, it is more convincingly demonstrated in the sagittal CT image.

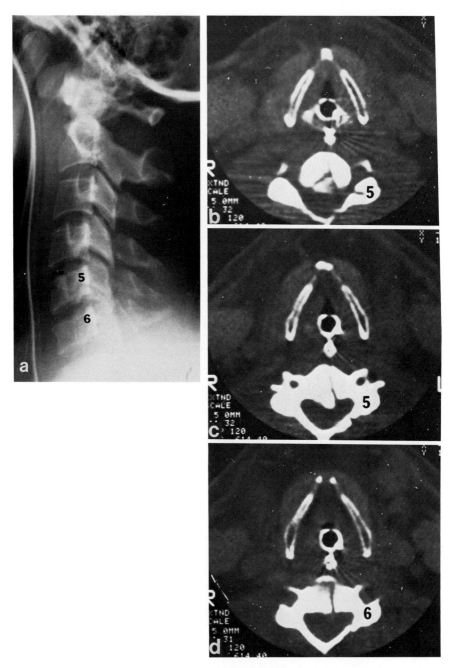

Figure 7.19. Lateral radiograph of the cervical spine of a young man who struck the top of his head on the bottom of a swimming pool at the end of a dive. The patient experienced instantaneous severe pain in the cervical region and was paralyzed from the shoulders downward. This examination was initially interpreted as being negative for fracture or dislocation. The minor irregularities of contour of the bodies of C_5 and C_6 were interpreted as normal variants or old post-traumatic changes, and the subtle posterior column abnormalities were not appreciated. Axial CT obtained because of the neurologic deficit and the disparity between the clinical and radiographic findings demonstrated a severely comminuted bursting fracture of C_5 with retropulsion of fragments into the spinal canal (*b* and *c*) and a minimally dispersed bursting fracture of C_6 (*d*).

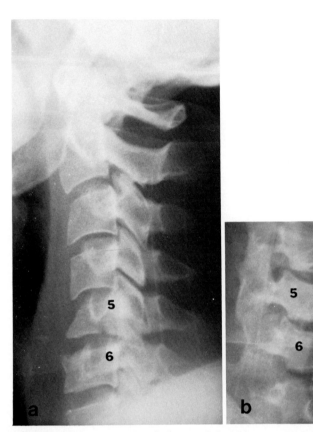

Figure 7.20.   Obvious bursting fracture of C$_5$ with very subtle bursting fracture of C$_6$. In the lateral projection (*a*), the "military" attitude of the cervical spine, comminution of the body of C$_5$ with retropulsion of posterior fragments, and the absence of distraction of the posterior column are all indicative of a bursting fracture. The very subtle contour changes of the body of C$_6$ are nonspecific and do not suggest an acute fracture. In the frontal radiograph (*b*), however, a vertical fracture (*arrowheads*) is present in the body of both C$_5$ and C$_6$. Axial CT of C$_5$ (*c*) demonstrates a bursting fracture with retropulsion of fragments into the spinal canal and bilateral fractures at the junction of the lamina and articular mass (*arrows*). Axial CT of C$_6$ (*d*) demonstrates a very faint fracture defect (*arrowhead*) of the centrum without dispersion or laminar fracture. Retropulsion of C$_5$ fragments (*arrowhead*) is best seen in the midline sagittal reformatted image (*e*), and the fracture of C$_6$ body (*arrow*) was best seen in the "off-lateral" sagittal reformatted image (*f*).

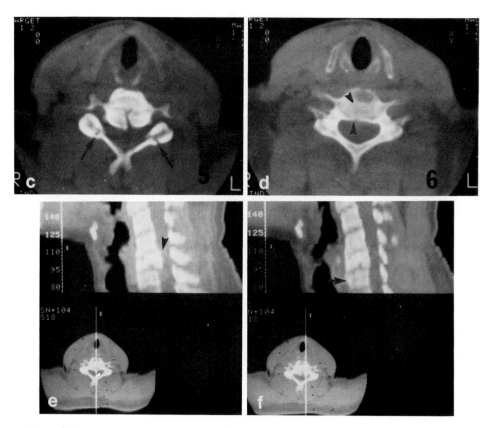

Figure 7.20.   *c–f.*

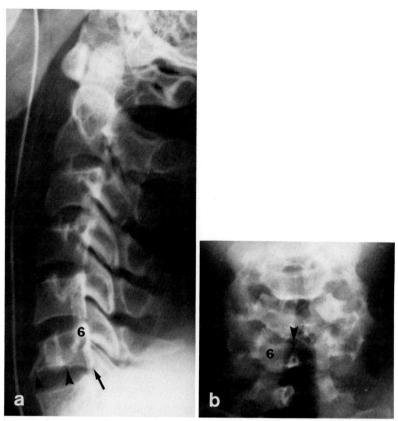

Figure 7.21. Very subtle bursting fracture of C_6 in lateral and frontal radiographs. In the lateral projection (*a*), the attitude of the cervical spine is normal, and, although the *configuration* of the body of C_6 suggests a simple wedge or compression fracture, none of the posterior column signs of a flexion injury is present. Further, close inspection of the C_6 centrum reveals comminution as evidenced by multiple fracture lines (*arrowheads*). Only the posteroinferior aspect of the body is very slightly retropulsed with respect to the posterior cortex of the body of C_7 (*arrow*). (This patient had no neurologic deficit.) The vertical fracture of the vertebral body (*arrowhead*), characteristic of the bursting fracture, is seen in the frontal projection (*b*). Absence of lateral displacement of the fragments and intact Luschka joints at the C_4–C_5 and C_5–C_6 levels indicate minimal dispersion of fragments. Because this patient had no neurologic deficit and because the plain-film signs of the injury were so clearly recorded and so typical of a bursting fracture, it was the opinion of the attending physician and the radiologists that additional radiographic examinations were unnecessary.

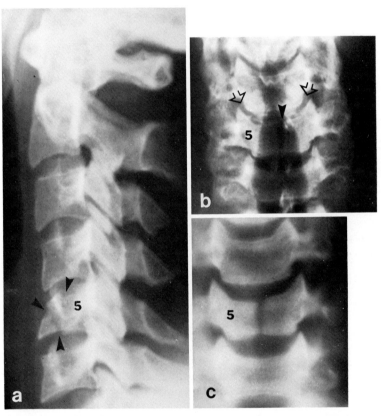

Figure 7.22. Bursting fracture of C_5 in lateral, frontal, and frontal polydirectional tomographic projections. In the lateral projection (*a*), the attitude of the cervical segments is that of the "military" position. The centrum of C_5 is comminuted with multiple fracture lines visible (*arrowheads*). Retropulsion of the posterior fragments is minimal if present at all. In the frontal plain radiograph (*b*), the typical vertical fracture (*arrowhead*) is evident. The Luschka joints at C_4–C_5 are slightly widened (*open arrows*) and at C_5–C_6 are slightly narrowed, indicating minimal lateral dispersion of fragments. The vertical fracture has been confirmed and more clearly delineated in the polydirectional tomogram (*c*).

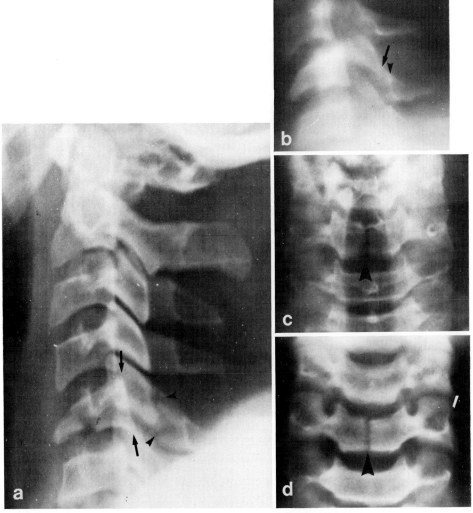

Figure 7.23.   Bursting fracture of C₅ in lateral projection (*a*) with retropulsion of posterior fragments (*arrows*) with respect to the posterior cortex of the bodies of C₄ and C₆ and laminar fracture (*arrowheads*) with caudad displacement of the laminae and spinous process. Polydirectional tomogram (*b*) demonstrates retropulsion of the body fragment(s), the laminar fracture (*arrow*) and the caudad displacement of the laminae and spinous process (*arrowhead*). Anteroposterior plain-film (*c*) and polydirectional tomograms (*d*) demonstrate the vertical vertebral body fracture (*arrowhead*).

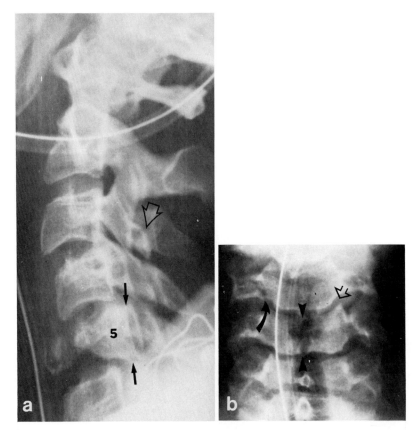

Figure 7.24.   Lateral radiograph (*a*) of a severely comminuted bursting fracture of C$_5$ with severe retropulsion of posterior fragments (*arrows*) relative to the posterior margins of the bodies of C$_4$ and C$_6$. The absence of signs of hyperflexion in the attitude of the cervical segments and the lack of distraction of the posterior elements is a fundamentally important observation. The frontal projection (*b*) demonstrates the characteristic vertical fracture of the vertebral body (*arrowheads*) and lateral displacement of the fragments with disruption of Luschka joints at C$_4$–C$_5$ (*open arrow*). This patient suffered a concomitant right articular mass fracture of C$_4$ (*curved arrow*).

included. To emphasize by repetition, the characteristic features of the bursting fracture that should be recognized on the lateral radiograph include (*a*) an essentially straight attitude of the cervical segments, (*b*) comminution of the vertebral body with retropulsion of its posterior fragments, and (*c*) the absence of signs of distraction of the posterior column, i.e., "fanning" and subluxation of interfacetal joints (Figs. 7.21–7.23).

The bursting fracture is considered mechanically stable in spite of the commonly associated myelopathy and laminar fracture because the interfacetal joints and posterior ligament complex are intact.

Chapter 8

Hyperextension Injuries

The family of hyperextension injuries results from a pure, or predominant, backward force delivered to the cervical spine, usually as a result of a vector force impacting on the mandible, face or forehead, or an abrupt deceleration injury in which the head and cervical spine are thrown into violent hyperextension. The specific type of injury depends on the direction and magnitude of the hyperextensive force. In this chapter, these injuries have been arbitrarily ranked from those with the least likelihood of associated neurologic damage (those that are the most stable at the time of injury) to those most likely to be associated with neurologic damage (those judged to be unstable at the time of initial injury). In this ranking, the hyperextension injuries include the following:

Avulsion fracture of the anterior arch of the atlas
Isolated fracture of the posterior arch of C_1
Extension teardrop fracture
Laminar fracture
Traumatic spondylolisthesis (hangman's fracture)
Hyperextension dislocation
Hyperextension fracture-dislocation

AVULSION FRACTURE OF THE ANTERIOR ARCH OF THE ATLAS

The avulsion fracture of the anterior arch of C_1 occurs when the hyperextension force in the upper cervical spine is transmitted through an intact anterior atlantoaxial ligament resulting in a transverse fracture of the anterior arch of C_1. This rare injury (110,111) is, of itself, not associated with either neurologic deficit or atlantoaxial instability. Radiographically, this fracture is best seen in lateral projection of the cervical spine and consists of a transverse defect, without sclerotic margins, in the mid or inferior portion of the anterior arch (Fig. 8.1). This fracture is associated with normal anterior atlantodental interval (AADI), intact posterior arch of C_1 and cervicocranial pre-vertebral soft tissue swelling. The characteristics of the fracture defect are optimally demonstrated by plain-film tomography. In frontal pro-jection, the avulsion fracture of the anterior arch of C_1 can be distin-guished from a high (type II) dens fracture because it extends beyond

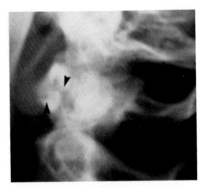

Figure 8.1.   Acute avulsion fracture of the anterior arch of C_1 (*arrowheads*).

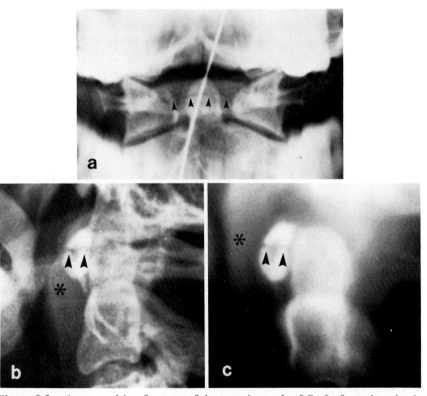

Figure 8.2.   Acute avulsion fracture of the anterior arch of C_1. In frontal projection (*a*), the lucent fracture defect (*arrowheads*) extends beyond the dens. The fracture line (*arrowheads*) and cervicocranial prevertebral soft tissue swelling (*) seen in the lateral radiograph (*b*) are more clearly demonstrated on the polytomogram (*c*).

the lateral margins of the dens and its position, with respect to the dens, will change following flexion or extension (Fig. 8.2). The fracture may be missed by computed tomography if the axial images are parallel to, but craniad or caudad to the plane of the fracture or if the plane of the fracture and the axial image coincide (Fig. 8.3).

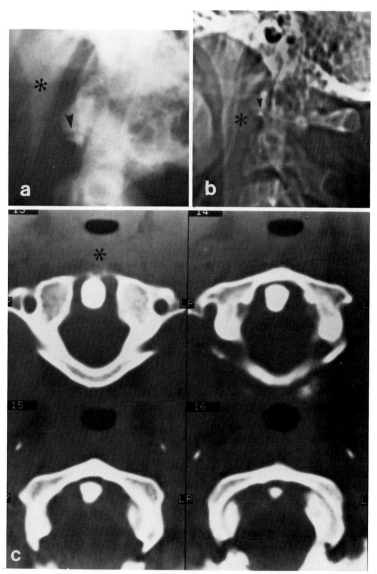

Figure 8.3. The acute avulsion fracture of the anterior arch of C_1 (*arrowhead*) seen on the lateral plain radiograph (*a*) and the CT "scout" view (*b*) was not recorded on the axial CT scans (*c*). Cervicocranial prevertebral soft tissue swelling (*) is clearly seen on each of these examinations.

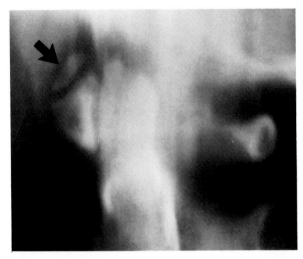

Figure 8.4. Polydirectional tomogram of ununited secondary ossification center of the superior margin of the anterior arch of C_1 (*arrow*). Note the smoothly sclerotic contiguous margins of the secondary center and the arch as well as the normal cervicocranial prevertebral soft tissues.

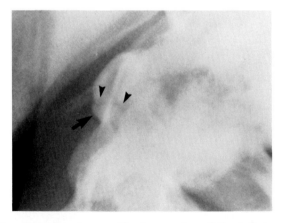

Figure 8.5. Ununited secondary ossification center of the inferior margin of the anterior arch of C_1 (*arrow*) is an incidental finding in this patient with facial trauma. The margins of the defect (*arrowheads*) are smoothly sclerotic and congruent. The soft tissue swelling is secondary to the midface fracture.

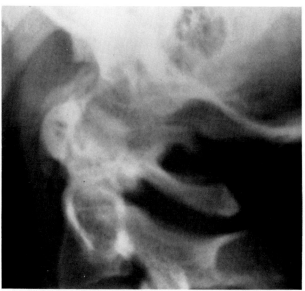

Figure 8.6. Ununited secondary ossification center of the inferior pole of the anterior arch of C_1 (*arrow*). The ununited center is round and smoothly corticated. The prevertebral soft tissues are normal.

Densely sclerotic or corticated margins, position, configuration, and the absence of prevertebral soft tissue swelling all help to distinguish ununited accessory ossification centers (Figs. 8.4–8.6) from the acute avulsion fracture of the anterior arch of the atlas.

ISOLATED FRACTURE OF THE POSTERIOR ARCH OF C_1

Fracture of the posterior arch of the atlas is a relatively common injury that results from the posterior arch of C_1 being compressed between the occiput and the heavy posterior arch of the axis during severe hyperextension (115). The fracture involves each side of the posterior arch posterior to the lateral masses and the transverse atlantal ligament. Because the fracture involves only the posterior arch of the atlas, it is a distinctly different lesion than the Jefferson fracture of the atlas.

Fracture of the posterior arch of the atlas may occur as an isolated fracture (Fig. 8.7) or in association with other types of cervical spine fractures (Fig. 8.8). Displacement of the fragments may be minimal, and oblique views may be necessary to identify the fracture.

The posterior atlantal arch fracture is not associated with either neurologic deficit or atlantoaxial instability.

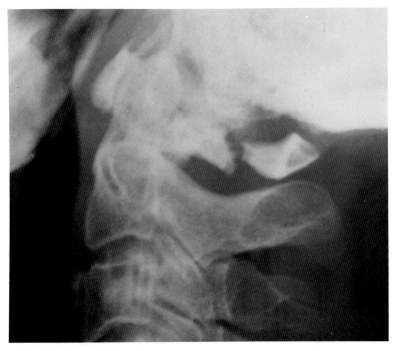

Figure 8.7. Isolated fracture of the posterior arch of the atlas. (From Harris, J.H., Jr.: Acute injuries of the spine. *Semin. Roentgenol.* 13:53, 1978.)

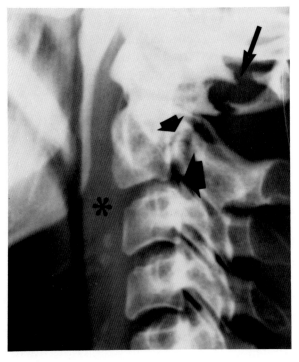

Figure 8.8. Fracture of the posterior arch of the atlas (*long arrow*) associated with traumatic spondylolisthesis (*arrowheads*). The asterisk (∗) indicates the prevertebral hematoma. (From Harris, J.H., Jr. & Harris, W.H.: *The Radiology of Emergency Medicine,* ed. 2. Baltimore, Williams & Wilkins, 1981.)

188

EXTENSION TEARDROP FRACTURE

The fracture involving the anterior inferior corner of the axis, resulting in a separate triangular fragment avulsed at the site of insertion of the intact anterior longitudinal ligament during hyperextension, has been designated the extension teardrop fracture by Holdsworth (21,47) and others (45,62,67). The extension teardrop fracture is more common in older patients with osteoporosis and degenerative disease of the spine. In osteoporotic patients, cervicocranial prevertebral soft tissue swelling is minimal (Fig. 8.9). When the extension teardrop fracture occurs in younger patients with normal mineralization, it is associated with obvious prevertebral soft tissue swelling that may extend into the lower cervical spine and the pharynx (Figs. 8.10 and 8.11), thereby resembling hyperextension dislocation. In this instance, the radiographic distinction between extension teardrop fracture and hyperextension dislocation must be based on the configuration of the separate fragment.

Radiographically, the extension teardrop fracture is characterized by the location and the shape of the fracture fragment. By virtue of the fact that the extension teardrop fracture is an avulsion fracture mediated through the intact anterior longitudinal ligament, the separate fragment constitutes the anterior inferior corner of the body of the axis, which is the site of insertion of this ligament. Typical of avulsion fractures, the plane of the extension teardrop fracture line is essentially perpendicular to the direction of its vector force.

The vertical height of the separate fragment equals or exceeds its horizontal (transverse) width, in distinction to the fragment frequently

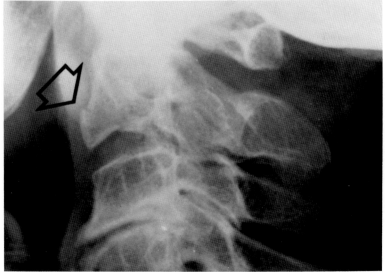

Figure 8.9. Extension teardrop fracture of the axis (*open arrow*).

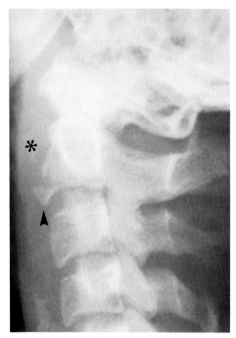

Figure 8.10. Extension teardrop fracture (*arrowhead*) of C₂ associated with diffuse prevertebral soft tissue swelling (∗) in a 20-year-old man.

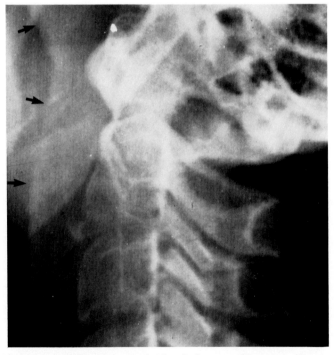

Figure 8.11. Severe, diffuse prevertebral soft tissue swelling extending into the oropharynx (*arrows*) associated with an extension teardrop fracture of the axis (*arrowhead*) in a 24-year-old woman who had no neurologic deficit.

seen in hyperextension dislocation in which the transverse diameter is greater than the vertical height.

Extension teardrop fracture is considered unstable in extension because the anterior longitudinal ligament is detached from the axis body, but is considered stable in flexion because the integrity of the posterior ligament complex and the interfacetal joints is maintained.

LAMINAR FRACTURE

Laminar fracture is a fracture of a cervical vertebra that involves primarily that portion of the posterior arch between the articular masses and the spinous process (Fig. 1.27) and results from compression of the lamina of one vertebra between those of the supra- and subjacent vertebrae during hyperextension. As previously described, when this fracture occurs in the atlas vertebra, it is referred to as the isolated fracture of the posterior arch of C_1. Although Effendi et al. (119) included the laminar fracture as one of the fractures of the ring of the axis, they failed to identify it as a discrete injury distinct from traumatic spondylolisthesis. This precise distinction is clinically appropri-

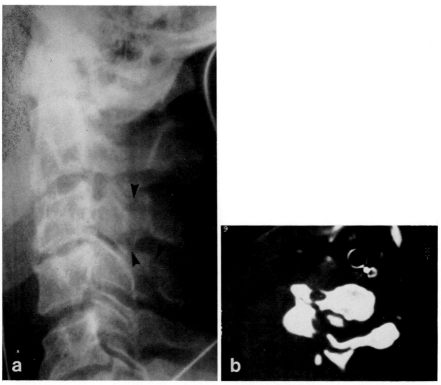

Figure 8.12. The comminuted laminar fractures of C_3 and C_4 (*arrowheads*) are very subtle and could be overlooked on the lateral plain radiograph (*a*). The axial CT scan (*b*) of C_4 establishes the fracture and defines the position of the fragments relative to the spinal canal.

ate because the laminar fracture occurs posterior to the pars interarticularis and the inferior articular facet of C_2 and is, therefore, not mechanically unstable as are Types II and III traumatic spondylolistheses. Thus, the laminar fracture of C_2 is analogous to the isolated fracture of the posterior arch of the atlas and to the laminar fractures of the lower cervical spine.

In the plain-film examination of the cervical spine, the laminar fracture is best seen in lateral projection (Fig. 8.12*a*) although it is commonly subtle and may be even more obscured by spondylosis. Plain-film tomography in frontal projection and axial computed tomography (Fig. 8.12*b*) are frequently required to demonstrate the laminar defect. CT is indicated in patients who have or are suspected of having a laminar fracture on plain-film radiography in order to confirm the diagnosis and to determine the position of fragments relative to the spinal cord.

The laminar fracture is mechanically stable since the anterior column and the interfacetal joints are intact. In the presence of a myelopathy secondary to cord involvement by laminar fragments, the laminar fracture should be considered unstable and the spine protected.

TRAUMATIC SPONDYLOLISTHESIS (HANGMAN'S FRACTURE)

Bilateral fracture of the *pars interarticularis* has been appropriately called "traumatic spondylolisthesis" (143) , "hangman's fracture" (2) and incorrectly termed, bilateral "pedicle" fracture of the axis (90,113,144).

The pedicles of C_2 are vague, ill-defined areas of the axis vertebra defined by Gray (10) as being "broad and strong, especially vertically where they coalesce with the sides of the vertebral body and the root of the dens. They are covered cranially by the superior articulating surfaces" (Fig. 8.13). The fracture of traumatic spondylolisthesis typically does not involve the anatomic pedicle. Instead, the most common site of this fracture is the pars interarticularis, i.e., the relatively thin portion of the articular mass between the superior and inferior articular facets of the axis, sometimes also called the isthmus (Fig. 8.14). Hence, "traumatic spondylolisthesis" most accurately describes this fracture.

"Hangman's fracture" may be an appropriate term for this fracture only because of the pathologic similarity of the accidental and the judicial fractures. The mechanism of the hangman's fracture, however, differs significantly by virtue of the distraction and shearing forces provided by the hangman's knot, which is unique to the judicial fracture.

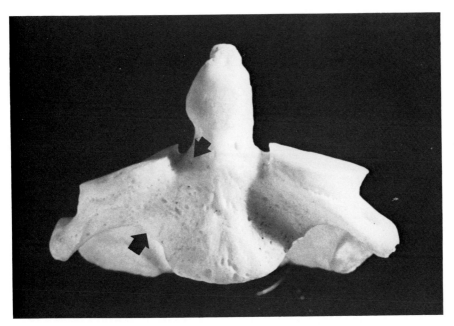

Figure 8.13. Frontal photograph of an axis vertebra. The area of the pedicle is indicated by *arrows*.

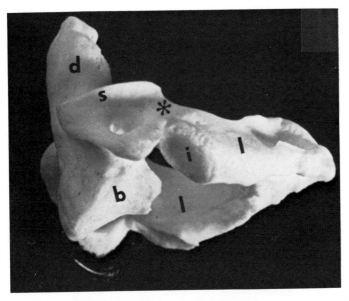

Figure 8.14. Axis vertebra photographed in obliquity from below upward in order to demonstrate the location of the pars interarticularis (∗) between the superior (*s*) and the inferior (*i*) facets. *d*, dens; *b*, the axis body; *l*, the laminae.

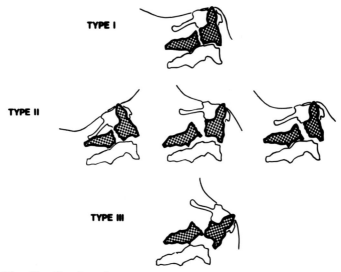

Figure 8.15. Classification of traumatic spondylolisthesis. (From Effendi, B., Roy, D., Cornish, B., Dussault, R. G., and Laurin, C. A.: Fractures of the ring of the axis: a classification based on the analysis of 131 cases. *J. Bone Joint Surg.* 63-B:319, 1981.)

In their article "Fractures of the Ring of the Axis," Effendi et al. (119) proposed a classification of isthmus fractures (Fig. 8.15) based on "the degree and type of displacement of the anterior fragment (the body of the axis) and the posterior fragment (the inferior facets of the axis) as expressed by the state of the disk space and of the articular facets at C_2–C_3." Although the ring fractures usually involve the pars interarticularis, the authors state that these fractures may also occur

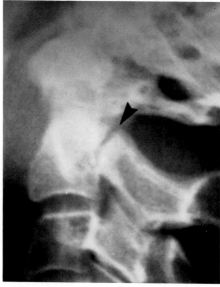

Figure 8.16. Typical type I traumatic spondylolisthesis with fracture through the pars interarticularis (*arrowhead*) and intact second intervertebral disk.

at the junction of the body and the articular mass, through the superior facet, the inferior facet, or the lamina. The bilateral fractures need not be symmetrical.

The Effendi classification (119) consists of types I, II, and III. Type I is defined as "isolated hair line fractures" of the axis ring "with minimal displacement of the body of C_2. The disk space below the axis is normal and stable" (Figs. 8.16–8.20). Type II is characterized by displacement of the anterior segment and an abnormal C_2–C_3 disk (Figs. 8.21–8.25). Type III fracture consists of anterior displacement of the anterior fragment with the body of C_2 in a position of flexion coupled with bilateral interfacetal dislocation of C_2–C_3 (Figs. 8.26 and 8.27).

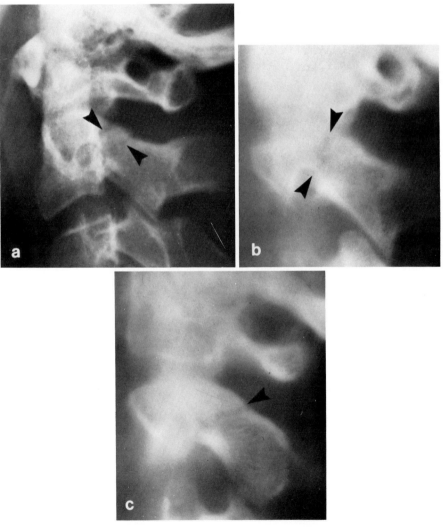

Figure 8.17. Subtle type I traumatic spondylolisthesis (*arrowheads*) in lateral radiograph (*a*). Polydirectional tomograms demonstrate the comminuted fracture (*arrowheads*) of the posterior aspect of the articular mass on the right (*b*) and the isthmus fracture (*arrowhead*) on the left (*c*).

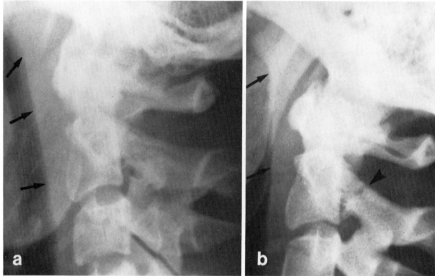

Figure 8.18.   The most prominent radiographic sign of this type I traumatic spondylolisthesis on the initial plain radiograph (*a*) is the cervicocranial prevertebral soft
tissue swelling (*arrows*). The soft tissue swelling (*arrows*) remains a prominent sign on
the true lateral radiograph (*b*) obtained minutes later and on which the pars fracture
(*arrowhead*) is clearly evident. In retrospect, the isthmus fracture is visible on the initial
examination (*a*).

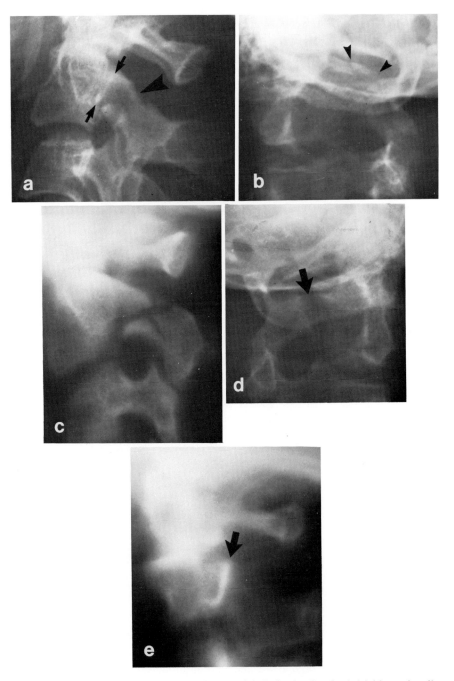

Figure 8.19. Atypical type I traumatic spondylolisthesis. On the initial lateral radiograph (a) a pars defect is evident (*arrowhead*) on one side and a vertically oblique cortical density (*arrows*) suggests a vertical fracture through the posterior aspect of the body of the axis on the opposite side. The left anterior oblique plain radiograph (b) and tomograph of the left side (c) confirm the comminuted isthmus fracture on the left (b, *arrowheads*). The right anterior oblique radiograph (d) and the polytomogram of the right side (e) confirm the extremely anteriorly situated fracture at the junction of the articular mass and the vertebral body (d, *arrow*). The vertical oblique density (e, *arrow*) is the posterior cortex of the centrum seen on the plain lateral radiograph (a).

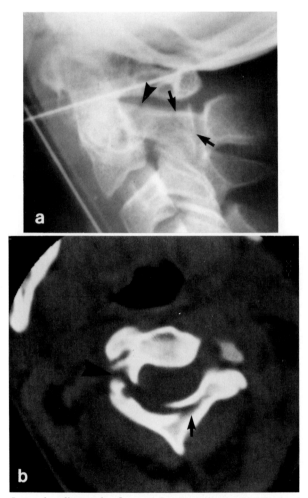

Figure 8.20. Lateral radiograph of a type I traumatic spondylolisthesis with an isthmus fracture (*arrowhead*) on one side and a posterior laminar fracture (*arrows*) on the other. The axial CT (*b*) confirms the isthmus fracture (*arrowhead*) on the right and the posterior laminar fracture (*arrow*) on the left.

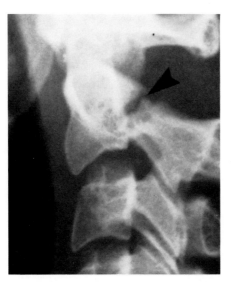

Figure 8.21. Type II traumatic spondylolisthesis with bilateral isthmus fractures (*arrowhead*) and disrupted second disk.

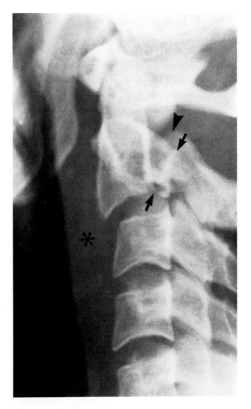

Figure 8.22. Type II traumatic spondylolisthesis with isthmus fracture on one side (*arrowhead*), fracture of the posterior aspect of the centrum on the opposite side (*arrows*), disrupted second intervertebral disk, and diffuse prevertebral soft tissue swelling (*).

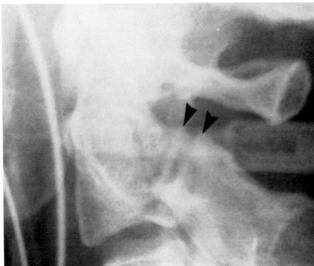

Figure 8.23.   Type II traumatic spondylolisthesis with each fracture through the posterior aspect of the pedicles as evidenced by parallel, vertically oblique densities of the posterior cortex of the axis vertebra (*arrowheads*). The second cervical disk is disrupted.

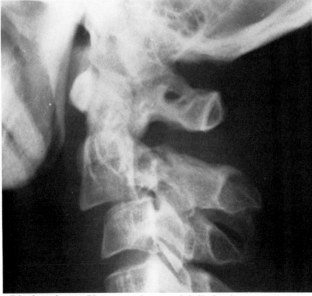

Figure 8.24.   Displaced type II traumatic spondylolisthesis.

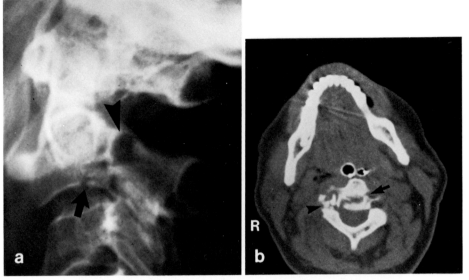

Figure 8.25. Lateral radiograph (*a*) of type II traumatic spondylolisthesis with an isthmus fracture on one side (*arrowhead*) and a fracture through the posterior aspect of the centrum on the other (*arrow*). The axial CT (*b*) demonstrates the axis body component (*arrow*) on the left and the comminuted isthmus and articular mass fracture that extends into the transverse process (*arrowhead*) on the right.

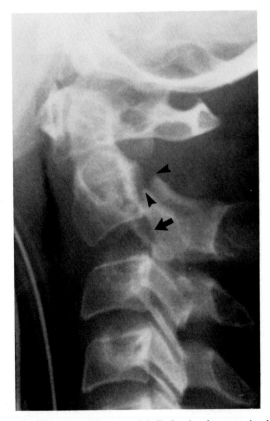

Figure 8.26. Type III traumatic spondylolisthesis characterized by bilateral pars interarticularis fractures (*arrowheads*), C_2–C_3 bilateral interfacetal dislocation (*arrow*) and disruption of the second intervertebral disk. Air in the retropharyngeal space is secondary to a mandibular fracture.

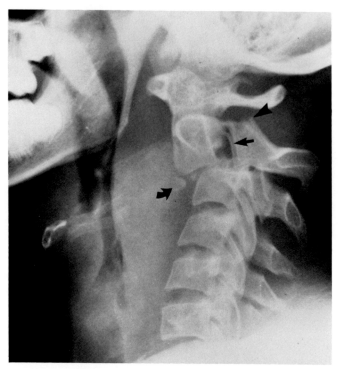

Figure 8.27. Type III traumatic spondylolisthesis with bilateral pars interarticularis fractures (*arrowhead*), bilateral interfacetal dislocation (*arrow*), disrupted second intervertebral disk, anteriorly displaced axis centrum, extension teardrop fracture of C_2 (*curved arrow*), and massive prevertebral soft tissue swelling. This young man, riding a trail bike, was caught across the neck by a wire stretched between two poles. The only neurologic deficit was bilateral upper extremity paresthesias that subsided spontaneously.

Traumatic spondylolisthesis is most commonly the result of a motor vehicle accident, although it may be caused by any type of abrupt deceleration at a high rate of speed such as a cyclist being caught by the neck while riding under a tightly stretched wire or clothesline. Initial hyperextension of the cervicocranium with, in certain instances, "rebound" flexion following dissipation of the initial hyperextension vector force is the most commonly accepted (16,24,53,101), although Sherk and Howard (168) report a single case of traumatic spondylolisthesis caused by "axial compression with flexion." More recently, Levine et al. (146) have refined the Effendi (119) classification and postulated different mechanisms of injury for each of these types of traumatic spondylolisthesis: type I, hyperextension-axial loading; type II, initial hyperextension-axial loading followed by severe flexion; type IIa, flexion-distraction; and type III, flexion-compression. Cornish (118), based on location and orientation of the posterior column fractures, operative findings, and autopsy dissections and experiments, postulated that a hyperextension-axial loading vector force causes traumatic spondylolisthesis. Effendi et al. (119)

have been credited by others (146) as attributing traumatic spondylolisthesis to the hyperextension-axial loading mechanism of injury when, in fact, Effendi et al. (119) stated: "These vertical compression forces are mainly secondary to violent hyperextension of the cervical spine." This vertical compression of the posterior column is simply reciprocal to the distraction of the anterior column caused by a hyperextension vector force. It is not the same axial loading force that causes the Jefferson bursting fracture and the bursting fracture of the lower cervical spine. The mechanism of the types I and II traumatic spondylolisthesis is more practically, pragmatically, and simply expressed as hyperextension of the cervicocranium, with the magnitude of force probably being greater in type II than type I and the compression of the posterior column recognized as inherent in the hyperextension rather than as a discrete second force vector. Effendi et al. (119) , and Levine et al. (146) ascribe type III traumatic spondylolisthesis to initial hyper*flexion* at the instant of abrupt deceleration (producing the interfacetal dislocation) followed by rebound extension (producing the isthmus fracture). Francis et al. (144) and Francis and Fielding (169) attribute traumatic spondylolisthesis, regardless of type, to hyperextension with posterior column compression ("axial loading") integral to the hyperextension. These authors, and others (118,167,146,119) cite the frequent association of posterior arch fractures of C_1 (Fig. 8.8) and C_3 and avulsion fractures of C_2 (Fig. 8.28)

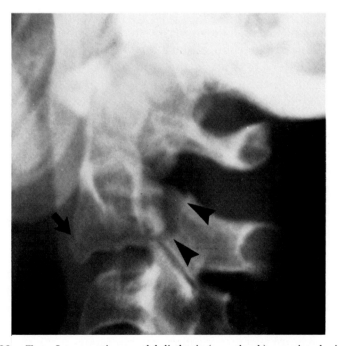

Figure 8.28. Type I traumatic spondylolisthesis (*arrowheads*) associated with extension teardrop fracture of the axis (*arrow*).

and C_3 as further evidence for hyperextension as the mechanism of injury.

In their review of 143 patients with fracture of the posterior arch of the axis, Effendi et al. (119) reported that 19 (14%) had associated injuries, of which eight were fractures of the posterior arch of C_1 (Fig. 8.8) and two were fractures of the dens. The remainder were randomly distributed among the lower cervical vertebrae.

Unless there is a distraction component at the time of injury, neurologic deficits associated with traumatic spondylolisthesis are usually minimal and transient because the anteroposterior diameter of the cord occupies only approximately one-third of the anteroposterior diameter of the canal at the C_2 level and because the bilateral posterior arch fractures produce "autodecompression" of the spinal canal. For these reasons, and contrary to the cord injury inherent in judicial hanging, the cord is "spared" in accidental traumatic spondylolisthesis.

HYPEREXTENSION DISLOCATION

Hyperextension dislocation is a poorly understood member of the hyperextension family of injuries because, although intervertebral dislocation occurs at the time of injury, the dislocation reduces spontaneously following dissipation of the causative force, resulting in the seemingly paradoxical situation of "hyperextension dislocation" when a dislocation is not present radiographically. Further, until the recent article by Edeiken-Monroe et al. (16), no critical analysis of the radiographic signs of this specific injury existed. It is not surprising, therefore, that hyperextension dislocation (HD) has been mistakenly described in older literature as the syndrome of the paralyzed patient with a normal-appearing cervical spine (109,121,23).

Hyperextension dislocation is caused by a straight backward or backward and upward force without a downward (or compressive) component which results in the following triad of signs: (*a*) soft tissue (or skeletal) injury of the midface or forehead, (*b*) some degree of the acute central cervical cord syndrome, and (*c*) diffuse prevertebral soft tissue and normally aligned cervical vertebrae on the lateral radiograph.

The pathology of HD is illustrated in Figure 8.29. The impacting force drives the head and upper cervical spine into hyperextension and the anterior column of the spine rotates upward and backward around the reciprocally compressed posterior column which serves as the fulcrum. With continued force, the anterior longitudinal ligament is ruptured and the intervertebral disk is either disrupted horizontally or detached from the inferior end-plate of the dislocated vertebral body. In the latter instance, as illustrated in Figure 8.29, the Sharpey's fibers (Fig. 8.30) remain intact, causing an avulsion fracture of the

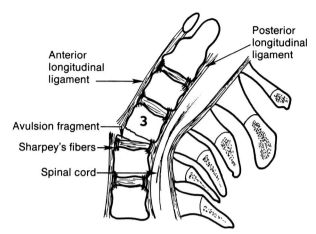

Figure 8.29. Schematic representation of hyperextension dislocation of C_3 illustrating the frequently associated avulsion fracture fragment arising from the anterior aspect of the inferior end-plate of the vertebral body. (From Edeiken-Monroe, B., Wagner, L.K., and Harris, J.H., Jr.: Hyperextension dislocation of the cervical spine. *AJNR* 7:135, 1986.)

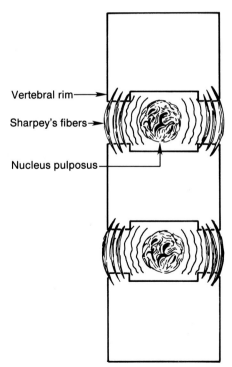

Figure 8.30. Schematic representation of the Sharpey fibers to the vertebral rim, which is the site of origin of the avulsion fracture of the anterior aspect of the inferior end-plate seen in approximately two-thirds of patients with hyperextension dislocation. (From Edeiken-Monroe, B., Wagner, L.K., and Harris, J.H., Jr.: Hyperextension dislocation of the cervical spine. *AJNR* 7:135, 1986.)

anterior aspect of the inferior end-plate. Further posterior displacement of the involved vertebra results in stripping of the posterior longitudinal ligament from the subjacent vertebral body. Posterior displacement of the dislocated vertebra results in the cervical cord being pinched anteriorly by the posterior cortex of the vertebral body and posteriorly by the dura, ligamentum flavum, and laminae. This compression results in the acute central cervical cord syndrome. With dissipation of the vector force, the dislocation spontaneously reduces.

The pathophysiology of HD illustrated and described above, and the term "hyperextension dislocation" were first pathologically established by Taylor and Blackwood (23) in 1948, although the same hypothesis and term used to describe the injury had been promulgated as early as 1920 by Wilson and Cochran (150).

The importance of recognizing HD as a specific, discrete injury and the acceptance, by Radiology, of the term used to describe it which is so well established in Orthopaedics and Neurosurgery justifies a concise, but comprehensive, review of the literature pertinent to hyperextension dislocation.

The patient reported by Taylor and Blackwood (23) in 1948 suffered an acute injury of the cervical spine "in which damage to the cervical part of the spinal cord appears without radiographic evidence of vertebral injury or displacement." Autopsy of this patient "revealed that the anterior longitudinal ligament was ruptured between the sixth and seventh cervical vertebrae, the column had been torn through by detachment of the intervertebral disk from the lower surface of the sixth vertebral body. The upper segment of the column, carrying with it the intact posterior longitudinal ligament, could be displaced backwards on the lower segment with great ease, the disk remaining attached to the upper surface of the 7th vertebra and the posterior longitudinal ligament being lifted from its posterior surface." In discussing this patient Taylor and Blackwood (23) stated: "A backward thrust applied through the head does cause dorsal *dislocation* or fracture at the lower levels of the cervical spine" and that injury causing the syndrome of a paraplegic patient with normally aligned, intact cervical vertebrae is "extension *dislocation* with immediate spontaneous reduction."

The identical combination of clinical, radiographic, and autopsy findings was described in four additional patients included in a study of 45 patients with hyperextension injury of the cervical spine reported by Marar (109) in 1974. As part of his study, Marar demonstrated that the application of a "backward rotation" force with simultaneous "strong posterior displacement (shearing) force" upon the head and neck of cadavers produces "definite backward subluxation."

One of six patients, all over 60 years of age, reported by Borovich et al. (104) developed acute cervical spinal cord syndrome subsequent to a fall. The lateral cervical radiograph was negative for fracture or dislocation. The patient died; at autopsy it was noted that the anterior longitudinal ligament was torn, the disk was disrupted horizontally, and the posterior longitudinal ligament was avulsed from the posterior aspect of the subsequent vertebra, i.e., hyperextension dislocation.

The pathologic lesion of hyperextension dislocation seen at autopsy by Taylor (56), Marar (109), and Borovich et al. (104), has been produced in anesthetized monkeys by MacNab (108,105) and Gosch et al. (54).

Even prior to the cadaver and animal research cited above, earlier authors had postulated just such an injury. Extension (hyperextension) *dislocation* of the cervical spine was first described by Wilson and Cochran in 1920 (150). In 1941, Mixter (151) hypothesized such a case by stating that "posterior *dislocation* is rare on account of the strong supporting structures, and, if it does occur, I believe that *spontaneous reduction might easily take place.*"

Post-traumatic tetraplegia without cervical fracture or dislocation was explained by Courville (147) and Watson-Jones (148) by the "recoil theory," defined as "momentary extreme vertebral *dislocation* causing cord damage with immediate spontaneous reduction of the *dislocation.*" Pancoast and Pendergrass (149) defined the recoil theory as "sudden massive *dislocation* of a vertebral body, which then reduces itself by antagonistic muscle action."

Forsyth (121) referred to this injury as hyperextension dislocation, while Gehweiler, et al. (46) referred to it as "hyperextension sprain (momentary dislocation) with fracture" and Braakman and Penning (45) as "hyperextension sprain."

Hyperextension dislocation is clinically and pathologically distinct from the injury described by Taylor in his article "The Mechanism of Injury to the Spinal Cord in the Neck without Damage to the Vertebral Column." (56) Taylor described a 67-year-old man who fell forward onto his face and was immediately quadriplegic with sensory loss from C_7. Cervical spine radiographs revealed only "senile degenerative changes." The patient died 9 days post injury from a urinary infection. At autopsy, the cervical spine was removed *en bloc*. The anterior longitudinal ligament was intact as were all of the intervertebral disks, joints, and ligaments. Histologically, the posterior columns were grossly destroyed with interruption and fragmentation of the nerve fibers. The damage extended anteriorly but with far less gliosis and no interruption of the nerve fibers. Taylor concluded that this injury was caused by hyperextension and that the cord was struck from behind. Subsequent cadaver, postmyelographic experiments demonstrated that, in hyperextension, a series of posterior indentations at the level of the interlaminar spaces narrows the canal by as much as 30%. The indentations represent the inbulging of the ligamentum flavum and dura.

Five of the six patients reported by Borovich et al. (104) (referred to above) had varying degrees of cervical spondylosis. One of them died after repeated falls. The four survivors all experienced some degree of neurologic recovery. In these patients, the central cord syndrome is best explained by the pinching of the osteophytes anteriorly and the inbulging dura and ligamentum flavum posteriorly. The case described by Taylor (56) and four of the six described by Borovich et al. 104) do not meet the pathologic, clinical, or radiographic criteria of hyperextension dislocation. They represent, instead, post-traumatic acute central cervical cord syndrome secondary to cord compression during hyperextension in patients with only cervical osteophytosis and *no musculoskeletal injury*. This phenomenon is called the "Taylor mechanism" and differs from HD by the absence of any radiographic abnormality of the cervical spine except the degenerative disease. Specifically, in the "Taylor mechanism," the cervical prevertebral soft tissues are normal.

Edeiken-Monroe et al. (16) have described the radiographic signs of HD in the adult as, (*a*) diffuse prevertebral soft tissue swelling with normally aligned cervical vertebrae (Fig. 8.31) present in all patients and the only signs present in 30% of their series of 20 patients, (*b*) an avulsion fracture rising from the anterior aspect of the inferior endplate of the dislocated vertebra (Fig. 8.32) (65%), (*c*) widening of the disk space ("increased height" (Fig. 8.33)), and (*d*) a vacuum disk (Fig. 8.34), each occurring in 15% of their patients.

The cervical prevertebral soft tissue swelling is diffuse in all patients in whom the ring apophyses are fused and extends from the thoracic inlet to the clivus. In 50% of patients reported by Edeiken-Monroe et al. (16), the prevertebral soft tissue swelling was more then twice the normal (eg., 4 mm at 72 inches and 7 mm at 40 inches) soft tissue width anterior to the body of C_3, regardless of the target-film distance.

In patients in whom the ring apophysis is ununited and in whom the paraspinous ligaments are more elastic, it is reasonable to assume that the dense, inelastic Sharpey fibers avulse the ring apophysis with less hyperextension force than is required to disrupt the anterior longitudinal ligament. Consequently, avulsion of the ring apophysis indicates the same mechanism of injury that produces a hyperextension dislocation. These patients usually may have no neurologic deficit, suggesting that complete dislocation does not occur. Prevertebral soft tissue swelling is localized and limited (Fig. 8.35).

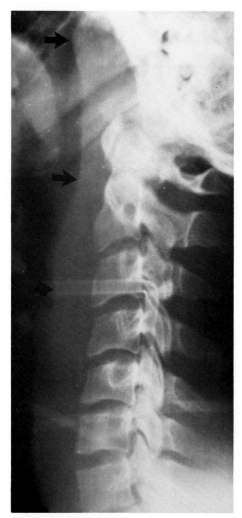

Figure 8.31. Hyperextension dislocation characterized by intact cervical vertebrae and diffuse prevertebral soft tissue swelling (*arrows*) extending throughout the cervical region and into the nasopharynx.

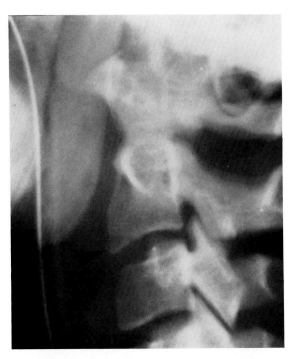

Figure 8.32. Hyperextension dislocation with avulsion fracture (*arrowhead*) of the anterior aspect of the inferior end-plate of C$_2$. The transverse diameter of the separate fragment is greater than its vertical height, characteristic of the fracture associated with hyperextension dislocation in approximately two-thirds of patients.

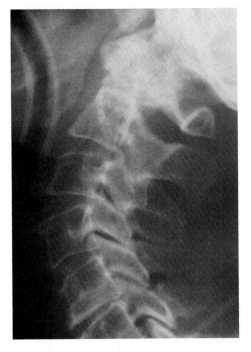

Figure 8.33. Hyperextension dislocation of C$_3$ with increased height of the third intervertebral disk space (*arrow*).

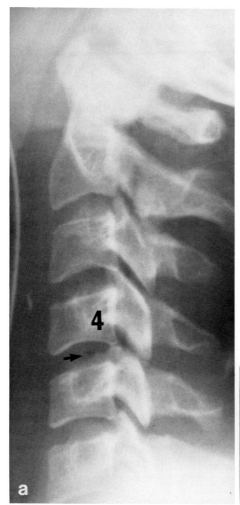

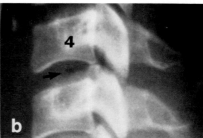

Figure 8.34. Hyperextension dislocation of C_4 with a vacuum defect (*arrow*) in the fourth intervertebral disk. *a* demonstrates the straightened attitude of the intact cervical vertebrae and diffuse prevertebral soft tissue swelling. The vacuum defect (*arrow*) is seen in *a* and a close-up in *b*.

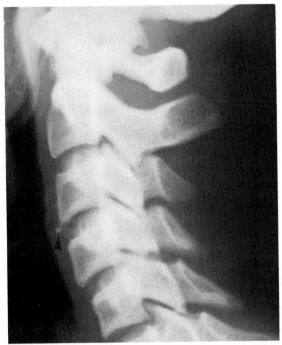

Figure 8.35. Hyperextension dislocation of C$_3$ marked by separation of its ring apophysis (*arrowhead*) and localized prevertebral soft tissue swelling. This patient was neurologically intact.

The avulsion fracture associated with HD has a characteristic location and configuration. The Sharpey fibers are the dense, tough elements of the annulus fibrosis that penetrate into the rim of the vertebral end-plate and attach the disk to the vertebral body. When, during hyperextension, the inferior end-plate of the dislocated vertebra separates from the superior surface of the disk, the Sharpey fibers remain intact and avulse the portion of the end-plate that earlier had been the ring apophysis, i.e., the rim. Consequently, the avulsion fracture fragment constitutes the anterior portion of the inferior end-plate of the vertebral body (Fig. 8.32) or, prior to its fusion with the centrum, the ring apophysis itself (Fig. 8.35).

The horizontal width of the avulsion fragment of HD exceeds its vertical height. This characteristic configuration distinguishes the fracture of HD from the extension teardrop fracture of the axis in which the vertical height equals or exceeds the horizontal width (Fig. 8.36).

Although some articles in radiologic literature have referred to HD by different terms (45,62,117), the autopsy findings and cadaver and animal experiments that substantiate posterior vertebral dislocation, together with the historic, traditional and current clinical acceptance of "hyperextension dislocation" make it the preferred designation of this unique member of the family of hyperextension injuries of the cervical spine.

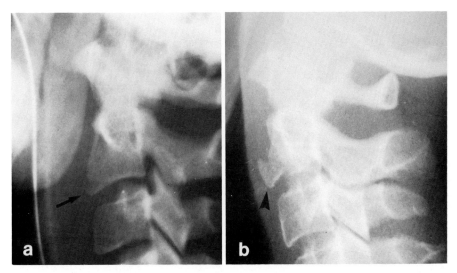

Figure 8.36. Typical fractures of hyperextension dislocation (*a, arrow*) and the extension teardrop fracture (*b, arrowhead*) of C$_2$. Characteristically, the horizontal width of the avulsion fracture of HD exceeds its vertical height, whereas the opposite is characteristic of the extension teardrop fracture fragment.

HYPEREXTENSION FRACTURE-DISLOCATION

The mechanism of injury of hyperextension fracture-dislocation postulated by Forsyth (121) is force delivered to the upper face or forehead, either eccentrically or with the head rotated, that forces the head and upper cervical spine into a backward and downward direction. Continued force results in severe attenuation and rupture of the anterior longitudinal ligament and impaction of the articular masses on the side opposite the direction of rotation or of the vector force, causing comminution of a subjacent articular mass (Fig. 8.37). As the force continues in its posterior and downward arcs, it assumes a forward direction (circular or "circus" movement), causing the supra-adjacent vertebra to translate anteriorly through the comminuted subjacent articular mass fracture while, on the contralateral side, the more forward force causes an interfacetal subluxation or dislocation. Disruption of the interfacetal joint by fracture on the side of impaction and by subluxation or dislocation on the opposite side permits forward translation of the vertebral body characteristic of this *hyperextension* injury.

The radiographic features of hyperextension fracture-dislocation are illustrated in Figure 8.38. In frontal projection, the normal uniform density and trabeculation of the lateral column and its seemingly smoothly undulating margin are disrupted on the side of the mass fracture by either fracture lines or by interfacetal joints made visible due to rotation or articular mass fragments. In lateral projection, the most obvious finding is slight anterior displacement of the involved verte-

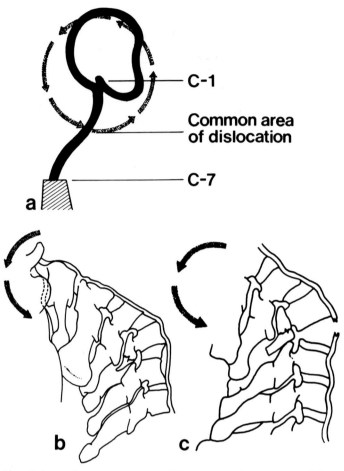

Figure 8.37. Schematic representation of hyperextension fracture-dislocation. The concept of a circular ("circus") vector force is illustrated in *a*. The pathophysiology of the early phase, with stripping of the anterior longitudinal ligament, distraction of the intervertebral disk and an articular mass fracture, is illustrated in *b* and a late phase, with disruption of the anterior longitudinal ligament and the intervertebral disk together with the articular mass fracture and interfacetal joint subluxation, is illustrated in *c*. (From Forsyth, H. F.: Extension injuries of the cervical spine. *J Bone Joint Surg* 46-A:1792–1707, 1964.)

bra. In hyperextension fracture-dislocation, the amount of forward displacement is usually 3–6 mm, i.e., less than in unilateral interfacetal dislocation but greater than in anterior subluxation (hyperflexion sprain). At the level of the articular mass fracture, the anatomy of the articular masses and interfacetal joints is completely disrupted. The inferior facet of the supra-adjacent vertebra may be driven upward (the "horizontal" facet (121)) or the facets may be so severely comminuted as to be unidentifiable (the "absent" facet). Fractures of the laminae and/or spinous processes may coexist. The articular mass fractures and interfacetal joint disruption of the impacted side and subluxation of the interfacetal joint ("perched" vertebra) on the opposite

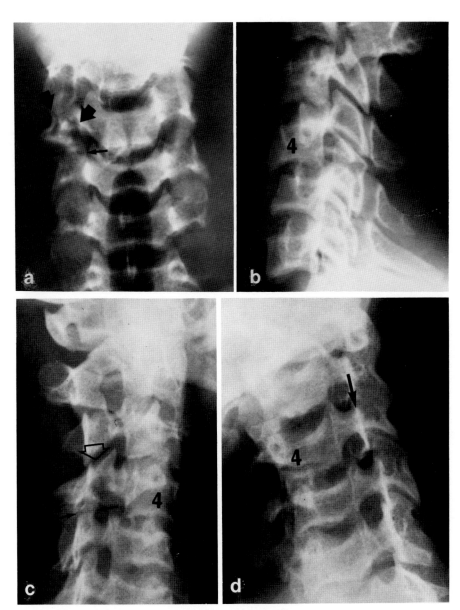

Figure 8.38. Hyperextension fracture-dislocation of C_4. In the frontal projection (*a*), the severely comminuted fracture of the right lateral mass of C_4 is indicated by the *large arrows* and the fracture of the superior facet of C_5 by the *small arrows*. In the lateral radiograph (*b*), the slight forward displacement of C_4 is evident. The right anterior oblique projection (*c*) demonstrates the severely comminuted fracture of the right lateral mass of C_4 (*open arrow*) and the compression and upward displacement of its inferior facetal fragments, producing the "horizontal facet." The *small arrows* indicate the fracture of the superior articulating facet of C_5. The opposite (left anterior) oblique radiograph (*d*) demonstrates the dislocation of the left interfacetal joint at the C_4–C_5 level. The left lamina of C_4 (*arrow*) is anterior to that of C_5.

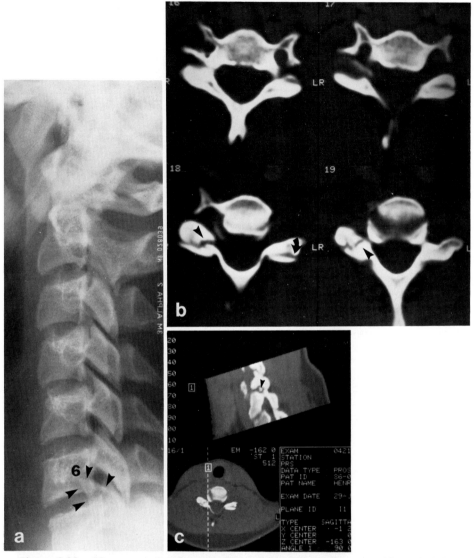

Figure 8.39. Hyperextension fracture-dislocation of C_6. In the neutral lateral plain radiograph (*a*), C_6 is very slightly, but definitely, anteriorly translated with respect to C_7, and a major displaced fracture (*arrowheads*) involves one of the C_7 articular masses. Axial CT (*b*) confirms the right articular mass fracture of C_7 (*arrowheads*) and subluxation of the left C_6–C_7 interfacetal joint (*curved arrow*). Sagittal reformation through the articular mass (*c*) demonstrates a small fracture fragment (*arrowhead*) in the intervertebral foramen. Three-dimensional reformation of C_6–C_7 seen from behind (*d*) shows the fracture of the superior aspect of the right articular mass of C_7 (*arrowheads*) and anterior displacement of the right articular mass of C_6. *e* is an oblique lateral view of the right articular masses of C_6 and C_7 as though seen from above looking downward. The anteriorly displaced superior fragment of the articular mass of C_7 (*) is clearly seen. The *arrow* indicates the anterior portion of the right superior articulating facet of C_7. The smooth surfaces at the top of the image represent the electronically transected surface of C_6. The inferior portion of its right articular mass (*am*) is impacted into the contiguous mass of C_7, resulting in the C_7 mass fracture. The right lamina of C_6 (*l*), its transverse process (*tp*) and foramen transversarium (*) are easily recognizable in 3-D reformation. In *f–h*, C_6 and C_7 have been electronically vertically

216

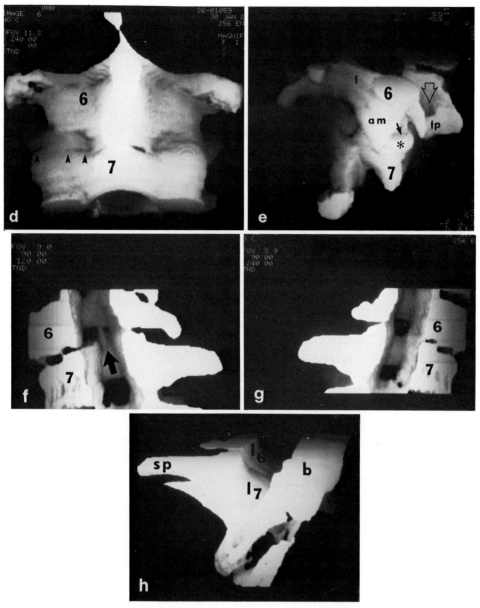

bisected and each hemivertebra is seen as though from within the spinal canal looking laterally. In f and g, the forward translation of C_6 is evidenced by the relationship of the body of C_6 to that of C_7, the posterior laminar line of C_6 anterior to that of C_7, and the spinous process of C_6 "perched" on that of C_7. The separate fragment (f, *arrow*) in the right intervertebral foramen is better seen in the 3-D reformation then on the sagittal CT (c). In h, the concept of "perching" as a sign of anterior translation is clearly illustrated in the vertically bisected image which has been rotated laterally and is viewed from below upward. In this image, where b is the anterior column (vertebral bodies), l the laminae, and sp the spinous process, the right lamina of C_6 (l6) can been seen situated directly above and slightly anterior to that of C_7 (l7). Normally, when viewed from this perspective, neither the inferior margin of the more cephalad lamina, normally lying above and behind its subjacent counterpart, nor the interlaminar space should be visible.

217

side are usually well seen in oblique projections. Polydirectional tomography, CT, or three-dimensional CT (Fig. 8.39) delineate the pathology of hyperextension fracture-dislocation to best advantage.

Hyperextension fracture-dislocation is considered unstable because the structural integrity of the lateral columns is disrupted by the articular mass fracture and the interfacetal subluxation or dislocation.

The practical importance of an awareness and understanding of hyperextension fracture-dislocation is that it must be recognized as one of the hyperextension injuries in spite of the *anterior* displacement of the involved vertebra. Anterior translation of a vertebra, or vertebral body, is typical of a flexion injury. If hyperextension fracture-dislocation is misinterpreted to be a flexion injury and treated by traction in extension, the treatment will, to some degree, reproduce the causative mechanism of injury.

Hyperextension fracture-dislocation is distinguished from a flexion injury by fracture lines involving the "lateral column" and its lateral margin in the frontal projection, by articular mass comminution, disruption of interfacetal joint anatomy, and the "horizontal" or "absent" facet signs in lateral projection. The comminuted articular mass fracture characteristic of hyperextension differs distinctly from the simple fractures of the facetal margins that may occur during hyperflexion. Therefore, minor anterior translation of a vertebra associated with signs of unilateral comminution of the articular mass(es) in the frontal and lateral projections indicates a hyperextension injury— specifically, hyperextension fracture-dislocation.

Chapter 9

Lateral Flexion

Lateral flexion (lateral bending, lateral tilt) (2,6,36,64,65,69,81,98,99) is either translation or canting of a vertebra in the plane of the X axis (Fig. 3.1). Lateral flexion rarely occurs as a pure or dominant vector force. When it does occur as an isolated mechanism of injury it produces the uncinate process fracture (Fig. 9.1). More commonly, lateral flexion occurs in association with another vector force—i.e., rotation at the atlantoaxial level to produce torticollis (Chapter 10, p. 247)— or as modifying some other dominant vector force such—as vertical compression producing an eccentrically displaced Jefferson bursting fracture (Fig. 7.9).

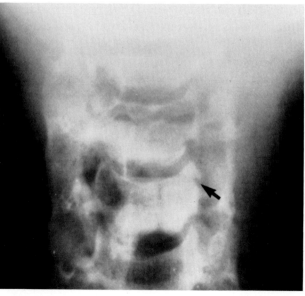

Figure 9.1. Fracture of the base of the left uncinate process (*arrow*) of a midcervical vertebra.

Chapter 10

Injuries of Diverse or Poorly Understood Mechanisms

This group of acute injuries of the cervical spine includes occipitoatlantal disassociation that may be caused by different (diverse) vector forces, dens fractures that are reported to be caused by a variety of different vector forces, and torticollis (atlantoaxial rotary displacement) that is associated with great variety of conditions, whose etiology and pathophysiology are enigmatic, and whose mechanism is poorly understood.

OCCIPITOATLANTAL DISASSOCATION

Occipitoatlantal disassociation (OAD) is a generic term that refers to abnormal separation or disruption of the occipitoatlantal (craniovertebral) junction and includes partial (subluxation) or complete (dislocation) disruption of the occipitoatlantal articulations.

The normal relationship between the occipital condyles and the superior articulating facets of the atlas is maintained by ligamentous structures that extend between the occiput and the atlas as well as between the occiput and the axis (see Chapter 1, p. 11). Consequently, vector forces that exceed the physiologic tolerance of these ligaments result primarily in ligamentous disruption or, less frequently, in avulsion of these ligaments from their sites of attachment at the craniovertebral junction.

Occipitoatlantal disassociation usually is a result of anterior translation (hyperflexion) of the skull with respect to the atlas, but may also be the result of distraction or posterior translation (hyperextension).

Because occipitoatlantal disassocation is usually a fatal injury (87), it is uncommonly encountered clinically. When frankly dislocated and unreduced, OAD is usually easily recognizable on a lateral radiograph of the skull or cervical spine (Figs. 10.1–10.4).

220

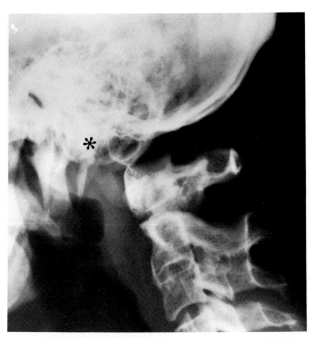

Figure 10.1. Fatal anterior occipitoatlantal dislocation with associated atlantoaxial rotary dislocation. The occipital condyles (∗) are anteriorly dislocated with respect to the superior facts of the atlas. The atlas has rotated about the dens and the anterior arch of the atlas is obscured by its anteriorly rotated right lateral mass. The posterior arch and the spinous process of the atlas are foreshortened due to the rotation.

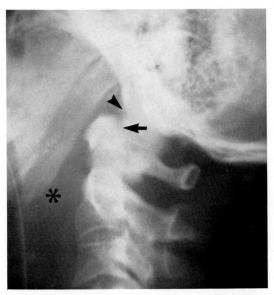

Figure 10.2. Posterior OAD. The tip of the clivus (*arrowhead*) is posterior to the posterior cortex of the dens (*arrow*) and diffuse, marked cervical cranial prevertebral soft tissue swelling (∗) extends to the clivus.

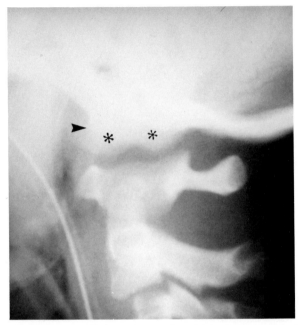

Figure 10.3. Simultaneous distracted anterior OAD and altantoaxial dislocation. The tip of the clivus (*arrowhead*) points to the superior margin of the anterior arch of the dens, and the occipital condyles (✻) are abnormally separated from the superior facets of the atlas. The atlas and axis are abnormally distracted. The presence of the endotracheal tube makes it impossible to evaluate the configuration of the cervico-cranial prevertebral soft tissue shadow.

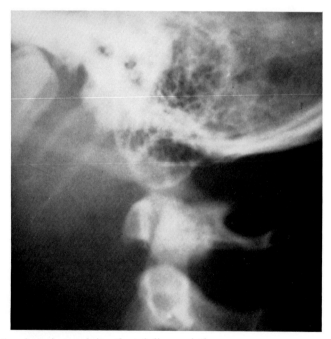

Figure 10.4. Anterior occipitoatlantal disassociation.

The radiographic signs of incomplete OAD or of partial simultaneous reduction of a frank OAD are usually subtle and extremely difficult to evaluate. In these instances, it is essential to recognize the secondary radiographic signs of craniovertebral disruption. Powers et al. (129) described the ratio of BC/OA (Fig. 10.5) as an accurate indicator of the presence or absence of *anterior* occipitoatlantal dislocation. The landmarks for determining the ratio are B, the basion (the anteriormost margin of the anterior rim of the foramen magnum— the tip of the clivus); C, the midvertical portion of the posterior laminal line of the atlas; O, the opisthion (the posterior margin of the foramen magnum); and A, the midvertical point of the posterior cortical surface of the anterior ring of the atlas. If the Powers ratio is less than 1.0, no *anterior* occipitoatlantal dislocation exists. If, on the other hand, the ratio is greater than 1.0, *anterior* occipitoatlantal dislocation is present. The strengths of this concept are that the ratio of BC/OA is an objective method of establishing subtle *anterior* OAD and that, being a ratio, its usefulness is unaffected by patient age or varying target-film distances. The weaknesses of the Power ratio concept are that it is commonly impossible to identify the opisthion and the posterior laminal line of C_1 accurately and the fact that the ratio has no application in the detection of posterior OAD. The latter observation becomes obvious with the realization that ratios less than 1.0, which are normal according to this concept, would be intrinsic with posterior occipitoatlantal dislocation.

Cervicocranial prevertebral soft tissue swelling (Fig. 10.6) in the absence of an obvious cervicocranial fracture or dislocation should prompt consideration of OAD (in addition to minimally displaced Jefferson bursting fracture, dens fracture, and traumatic spondylolisthe-

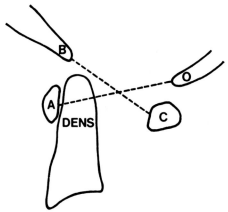

Figure 10.5. The Powers ratio is defined as BC/OA, where B is the basion, C the midpoint of the posterior laminar line of the atlas, O the opisthion, and A the midpoint of the posterior surface of the anterior arch of C_1.

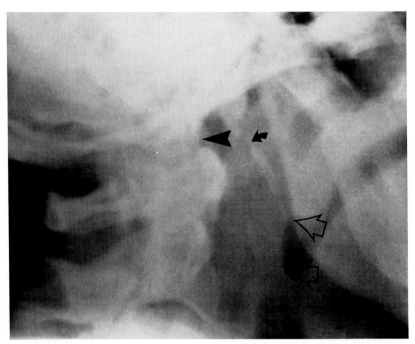

Figure 10.6. Anterior OAD heralded by marked cervicocranial prevertebral soft tissue swelling (*open arrows*) that extends to the skull base. The clivus (*arrowhead*) points to the posterior cortex of the anterior arch of the dens. Incidentally, one of the styloid processes is fractured (*curved arrow*).

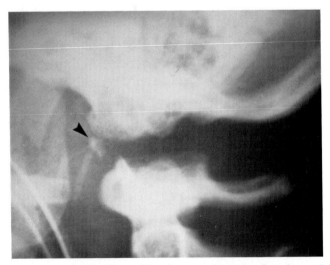

Figure 10.7.   Anterior OAD with avulsion fracture (*arrowhead*) at the occipitoatlantal junction.

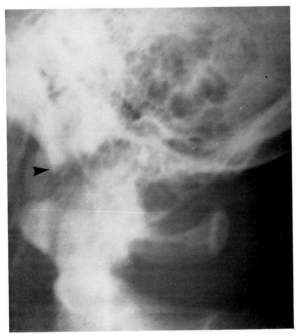

Figure 10.8. Anterior OAD evidenced by marked anterior displacement of the basion (*arrowhead*) with respect to the tip of the dens.

sis). Tiny fracture fragments at the occipitovertebral (Fig. 10.7) junction should be considered avulsion fractures indicating ligamentous separation from sites of attachment and, therefore, ligamentous instability at the occipitovertebral junction.

The tip of the clivus (basion) normally points to the tip of the dens. Werne (15) has established that this relationship is maintained regardless of the degree of flexion or extension of the skull with respect to the atlantoaxial articulation. Since the relationship between the basion and the tip of the dens is maintained by the same ligaments that maintain the occipitoatlantal articulation, it seems logical that anterior (Fig. 10.8) or posterior displacement of the basion with respect to the tip of the dens should reflect ligamentous disruption at the occipitoatlantal junction, i.e., occipitoatlantal disassociation. Preliminary studies (164) seem to support this hypothesis.

ODONTOID (DENS) FRACTURES

Fractures of the dens have been classified by Anderson and D'Alonzo (131) on the basis of the location of the fracture (Fig. 10.9). Type I, which is reported to be an oblique avulsion fracture of the tip of the dens at the site of attachment of the alar ligament, is an extremely rare injury. A current review of the English language literature disclosed

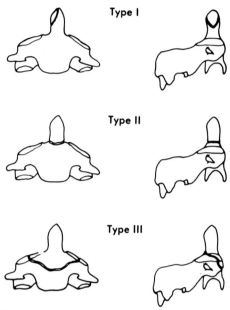

Figure 10.9. Classification of dens fractures according to Anderson and D'Alonzo (131).

only two proven cases of type I dens fractures in addition to the two reported by Anderson and D'Alonzo. A recent analysis of 25 dens fractures (133) and of an additional 50 patients with atlas fractures (164), including 24 dens fractures, failed to reveal a single type I fracture.

The type I dens fracture is generally considered to be stable and uncomplicated by nonunion. However, a more reasonable premise based upon the normal anatomy of the occipitoatlantal junction and the pathophysiology of the type I fracture, namely detachment of an alar ligament from the dens, is that the type I dens fracture is unstable and indicative of occipitoatlantal disassociation.

Because the Anderson and D'Alonzo type I dens fracture is so rare, several investigators (62,146,163) have proposed that the Anderson-D'Alonzo type I fracture not be considered a primary dens fracture, but a manifestation of occipitoatlantal disassociation and that dens fractures be classified only as "high" (Anderson and D'Alonzo type II) and "low" (Anderson and D'Alonzo type III).

"High" (type II) and "low" (type III) dens fractures may be caused by hyperflexion or hyperextension vector forces. The mechanism of injury in these instances is indicated by the obliquity of the fracture line and the position of the proximal (cranial) fragment (Figs. 10.10 and 10.11). In those instances where the dens is comminuted or the proximal fragment nondisplaced, the mechanism of injury cannot be deduced radiographically (Fig. 10.12).

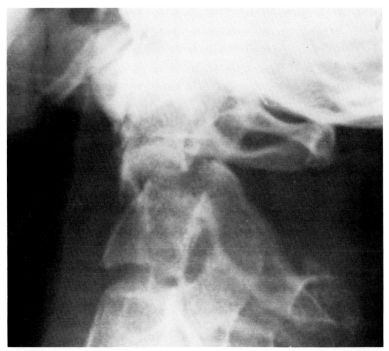

Figure 10.10 Low (type III) dens fracture with anterior translation and displacement of the dens.

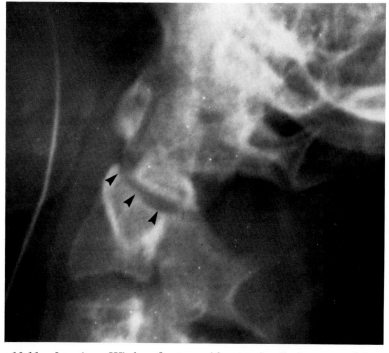

Figure 10.11. Low (type III) dens fracture with posterior displacement of the proximal fragment. The fracture line is indicated by the *arrowheads*.

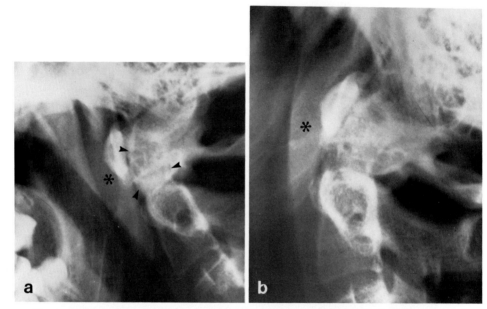

Figure 10.12.   Comminuted, nondisplaced high (type II) dens fracture. In the lateral plain radiographs obtained in flexion (*a*) and extension (*b*), multiple sites of disruption of the dens cortex (*arrowheads*) are evident. Change in the position of the dens with respect to the axis body indicates atlantoaxial instability. The cervicocranial prevertebral soft tissues (*) are swollen. Polydirectional tomography in frontal (*c*) and lateral (*d*) position confirm the comminuted, nondisplaced high dens fracture. The axial CT (*e*) is equivocal regarding the presence of a dens fracture. Three-dimensional CT images viewed from behind with the posterior arch of C_1 subtracted demonstrate the basilar dens fracture (*arrows*) in straight posterior (*f*), anteriorly rotated posteroanterior (*g*), and ROA (*h*) and LOA (*j*) projections.

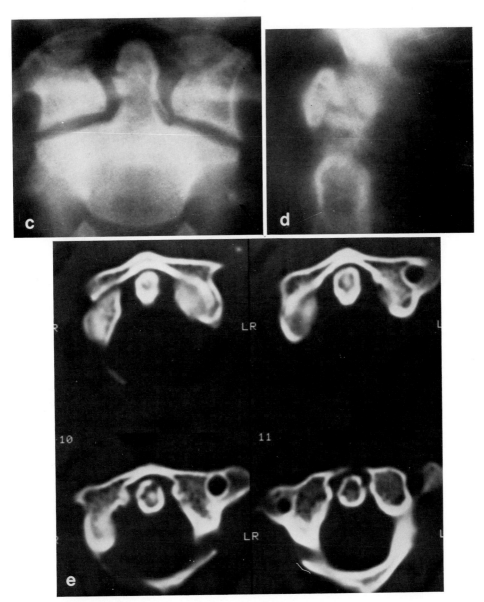

Figure 10.12. *c-e.*

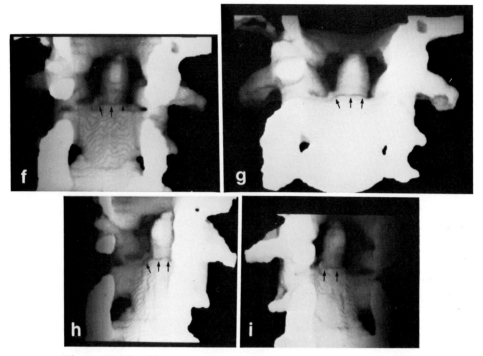

Figure 10.12.   *f-i.*

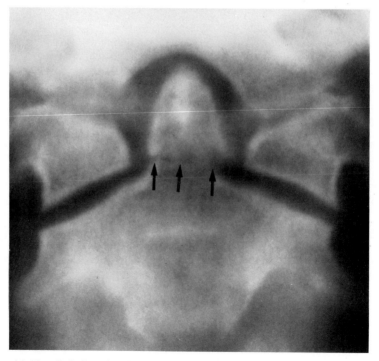

Figure 10.13.   Polydirectional tomogram of a high dens fracture. The fracture line (*arrows*) involves only the dens.

The "high" (II) dens fracture is limited to the odontoid process itself and typically involves the inferior portion of the dens. Radiographically, the high dens fracture is characterized by a transverse or obliquely transverse fracture through the lower portion of the dens. The fracture is confined to the dens only (Fig. 10.13). In lateral projection, acute high (and low) dens fractures are invariably associated with cervicocranial prevertebral soft tissue swelling (Fig. 10.14) which frequently is the most prominent radiographic sign of cervicocranial injury. The high dens fracture may be obscured by superimposed osseous structures in both frontal and lateral projections and, in these

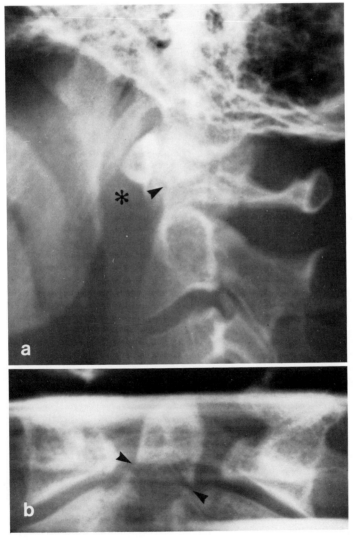

Figure 10.14. Diffuse cervicocranial prevertebral soft tissue swelling (∗) in the lateral radiograph (*a*) is the most striking radiographic sign of the subtle high dens fracture (*arrowheads*) confirmed by polydirectional tomography (*b*).

circumstances, plain-film tomography, panoramic zonography, or CT, particularly three-dimensional CT (Fig. 10.12), is required to establish or confirm the presence of the fracture defect. For reasons previously described, a high dens fracture oriented in the axial plane may not be demonstrated on axial CT images, but should be demonstrated on sagittal and coronal reformations (Fig.10.15).

In the frontal projection of the atlantoaxial articulation, the fact that the high dens fracture defect is limited to the dens distinguishes it from the avulsion fracture of the anterior arch of the atlas in which the fracture line extends laterally beyond the lateral cortices of the

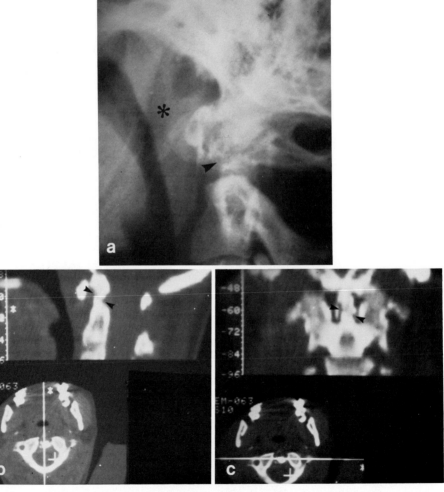

Figure 10.15. Comminuted, minimally displaced high dens fracture (*arrowheads*) seen in lateral projection (*a*). Note the diffuse cervicocranial prevertebral soft tissue swelling (*). The fracture is clearly delineated (*arrowheads*) in sagittal (*b*) and coronal (*c*) reformation.

dens (Fig. 8.2). The inferior cortex of the posterior arch of the atlas may produce a Mach effect simulating a high dens fracture. Typically, the Mach effect extends beyond the lateral margins of the dens and is superimposed on the lateral atlantodental intervals (Fig. 10.16) thereby excluding this lucency as a high dens fracture. If that observation cannot be made, simply repeating the open-mouth projection in a slightly different position will alter the relationship of this Mach effect to the dens while the position of a high dens fracture defect would remain unchanged.

In the lateral projection, the high dens fracture, unless frankly displaced, may be difficult to visualize because of the superimposition of the lateral masses of the atlas. Minimally displaced high dens fractures may be identified by disruption or "step-off" (Fig. 10.17) of the anterior or posterior cortex of the caudal portion of the dens. In lateral projection, the secondary sign of cervicocranial prevertebral soft tissue swelling is the most constant, and frequently the most striking, indication of a minimally displaced dens fracture of either type.

In appropriate clinical circumstances, and only under direct physician supervision, lateral flexion and extension views of the cervical spine may be used to confirm by abnormal motion of C_1 on C_2, the presence of a high dens fracture that is only suspected on the neutral lateral projection (Fig. 10.18). This technique is not advocated as a routine procedure because of the potential for producing, or aggravating, cord damage. Plain-film or computed tomography is the method of choice to confirm the presence of subtle dens fractures.

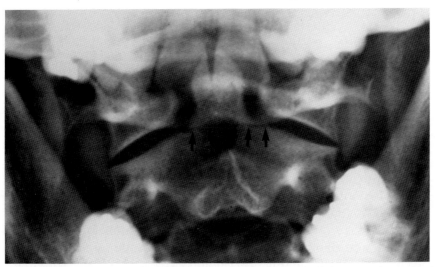

Figure 10.16. The superimposition of the inferior margin of the posterior arch of the atlas on the base of the dens results in a radiolucent Mach effect that closely simulates a fracture line (*arrows*).

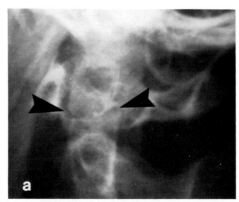

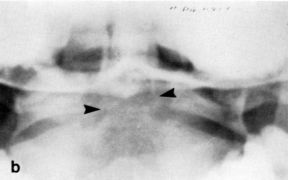

Figure 10.17. High dens fracture with minimal displacement and cortical "step-off." In the lateral projection (*a*), minimal anterior displacement of the cephalad fragment has resulted in both anterior and posterior cortical "step-off" (*arrowheads*). In the "open-mouth projection" (*b*), lateral cortical disruption is present at the base of the dens (*arrowheads*).

Because that portion of the dens fracture involved by the "high" fracture contains a relatively high amount of cortical bone, nonunion has been reported by Schatzker et al (152) to occur in 64% of dens fractures overall and nearly 100% of those with greater than 5 mm posterior displacement of the separate fragment. Both acute and ununited high dens fractures result in atlantoaxial instability because the proximal (cephalad) fragment and the atlas constitute a single unit. Ununited high dens fracture is called os odontoideum. Fielding (153) believes that the os odontoideum is post-traumatic in etiology, although nonfusion of the dens to the body of the axis has been observed in young children with no history of cervical spine trauma. Whether the os odontoideum is congenital or traumatic in origin is of little practical relevance. Its significance is that the os odontoideum is mechanically unstable (Fig. 10.19) and carries with it the potential of cord injury from relatively minor trauma.

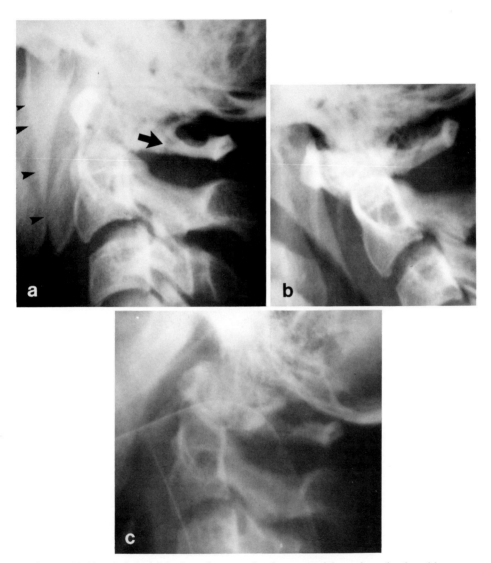

Figure 10.18.   Subtle high dens fracture in the neutral lateral projection (*a*) suspected on the basis of cervicocranial prevertebral soft tissue swelling (*arrowheads*) and loss of definition of the dens, itself. There is a concomitant minimally displaced fracture of the posterior arch of C_1 (*arrows*). Under physician controlled circumstances, gentle flexion (*b*) and extension (*c*) lateral radiographs demonstrate motion of C_1 with respect to the body of the axis, confirming the high dens fracture.

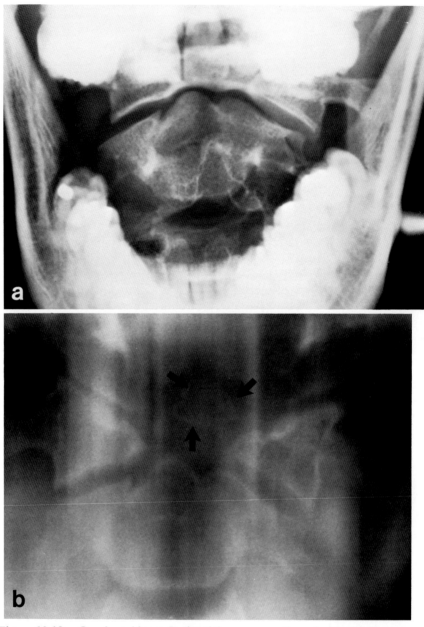

Figure 10.19. Os odontoideum. In the plain open-mouth projection (*a*), the separate ossicle is obscured by the superimposed incisor teeth and the anterior arch of the atlas. The appearance of the superior aspect of the body of the axis, however, suggests the presence of an os odontoideum by its smooth, corticated, lobulated margin. The separate ossicle (*arrows*) is visible in the frontal tomogram (*b*). In the lateral hyperextended radiograph (*c*), abnormal motion of C_1 with respect to the body of C_2 is clearly evident, indicating that the head, atlas, and ununited dens move as a unit with respect to the axis body.

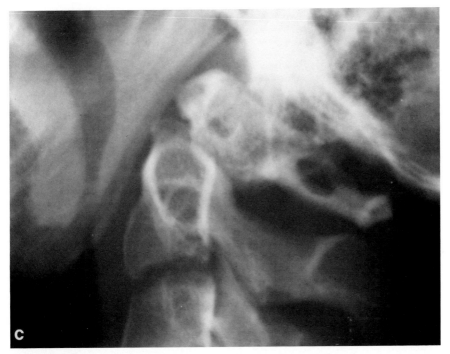

Figure 10.19. *c.*

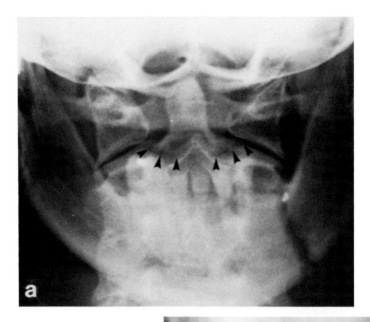

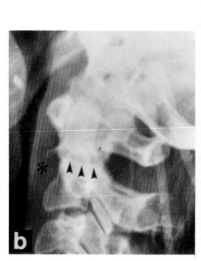

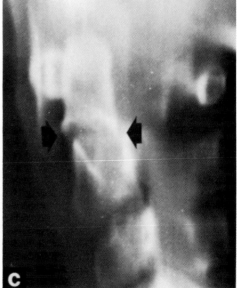

Figure 10.20.   Type III (low) dens fracture in a patient with multiple injuries, including a left mandibular fracture. The dens fracture line (*arrowheads*) is very subtle in both the open mouth (*a*) and lateral (*b*) projections. In the lateral radiograph, a thin bony fragment which arises from the dens, projects into the prevertebral soft tissues which are abnormally thickened (∗) by the associated hematoma. The fracture line (*arrows*) and displacement of the fragments are obvious in the lateral tomogram (*c*).

The "low" (III) dens fracture is not a fracture of the dens at all, but is actually a fracture of the superior portion of the axis body (Fig. 10.20) caudad to the junction of the dens and the axis centrum. As such, it involves an area of primarily cancellous bone and, consequently, almost always heals. Because the low dens fracture allows the dens, the atlas and the occiput to move as a unit, it is therefore considered to be mechanically unstable.

Radiographically, in the open-mouth projection, the low dens fracture extends in an inferiorly convex pattern from one superior articulating facet of the axis to the other. The configuration of the low dens fracture line resembles the drape of a mantle or cape across the shoulders (Fig. 10.21). The superior articulating facets are usually eccentrically involved, and their surfaces are disrupted and occasionally depressed (Fig. 10.22).

In the lateral radiograph, because of its course through the superior portion of the axis body, the low dens fracture disrupts the axis "ring" (133). The axis ring is an elongated, inferiorly tapered composite density (Fig. 10.23) comprised of the cortex of the junction of the pedicle and the centrum anteriorly, the cortex at the junction of the dens and body superiorly, and the posterior cortex of the axis body posteriorly (Fig. 10.24). In a review of 50 patients with dens fractures

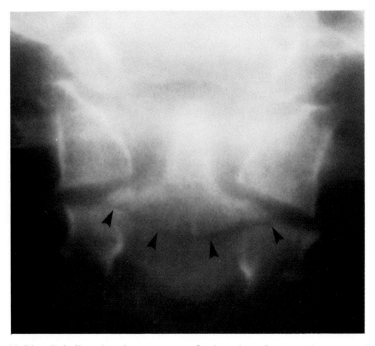

Figure 10.21. Polydirectional tomogram of a low dens fracture demonstrating the typical distribution of the fracture line (*arrowheads*).

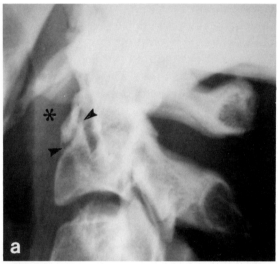

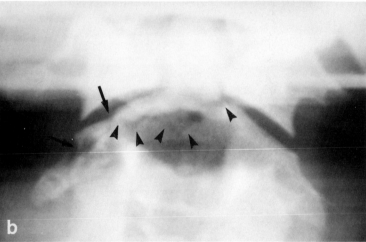

Figure 10.22. Low dens fracture characterized in lateral projection (*a*) by disruption of the axis ring (*arrowheads*) and cervicocranial prevertebral soft tissue swelling (∗). In the frontal polytomogram (*b*), the fracture line (*arrowheads*) extends eccentrically across the superior aspect of the axis body with comminution and depression of the right superior articular facet (*arrows*).

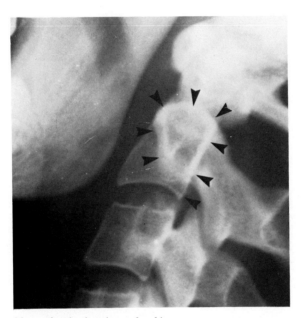

Figure 10.23. Normal axis ring (*arrowheads*).

(133), the axis "ring" was intact in all 22 patients with a high fracture and disrupted in all 28 patients with a low dens fracture. Disruption of the axis "ring" may be the only direct sign of a minimally or non-displaced low dens fracture in the lateral projection (Fig. 10.25). This is a particularly useful sign in those patients in whom, for whatever reason, the atlantoaxial articulation, and specifically the dens, cannot

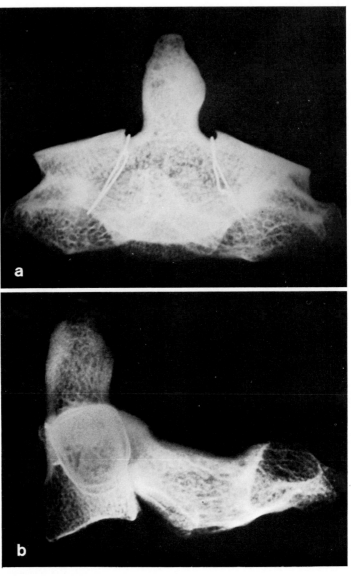

Figure 10.24   Radiograph of dried axis vertebra in frontal (*a*) and lateral (*b*) projections. The circumferential wires indicate those portions of the axis which constitute the ring.

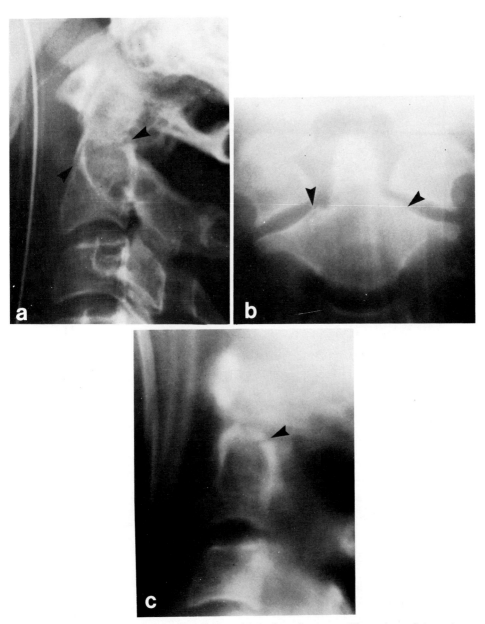

Figure 10.25 Subtle, minimally displaced low dens fracture. Disruption of the axis ring (arrowheads) in the lateral radiograph (*a*) is the only sign of the fracture. Cervicocranial prevertebral soft tissues cannot be evaluated because of the endotracheal tube. The fracture line (*arrowheads*) is confirmed in frontal (*b*) and lateral (*c*) polytomograms.

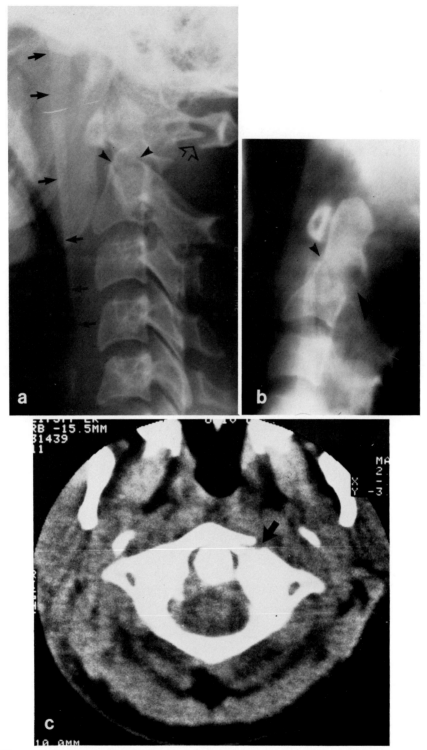

Figure 10.26. Low dens fracture associated with a Jefferson bursting fracture. In the lateral radiograph (*a*), the axis ring is disrupted (*arrowheads*) indicating a low dens fracture. The posterior arch of C_1 is fractured (*open arrow*) and the cervicocranial prevertebral soft tissues are abnormal from C_4 to the clivus (*arrows*). The lateral polytomogram (*b*) confirms the low dens fracture (*arrowheads*) and the axial CT scan demonstrates the C_1 anterior arch fracture (*arrow*).

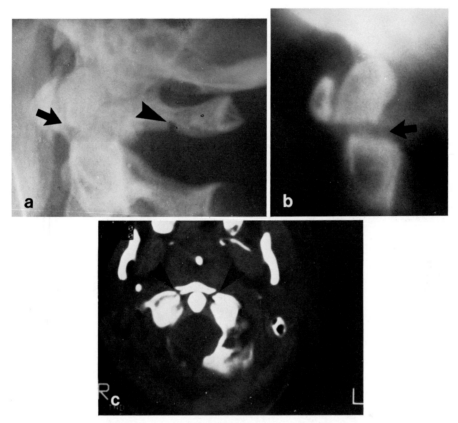

Figure 10.27. Anteriorly translated, posteriorly canted high dens fracture (*arrows*) associated with a Jefferson bursting fracture (*arrowheads*) in the neutral lateral plain radiograph (*a*), lateral polytomogram (*b*) and axial CT scan (*c*).

be visualized in frontal projection. As with high dens fractures, polydirectional tomography, panoramic zonography, and CT are useful to demonstrate subtle low dens fractures.

Dens fractures may be associated with Jefferson bursting fracture (Figs. 10.26 and 10.27) or occipitoatlantal disassociation (126), of the face or mandible (Fig. 10.20).

ACUTE TRAUMATIC ROTARY ATLANTOAXIAL DISLOCATION

Acute traumatic atlantoaxial dislocation is a rare injury (154–156) in which there is partial or complete derangement of the lateral atlantoaxial articulations associated with varying degrees of ligamentous injury at this level. Although "rotary" suggests a pure rotational vector force, it is physiologically not possible for a rotation of the atlas to occur on the axis without some element of lateral tilt; therefore, the mechanism of injury of acute traumatic atlantoaxial dislocation is unclear.

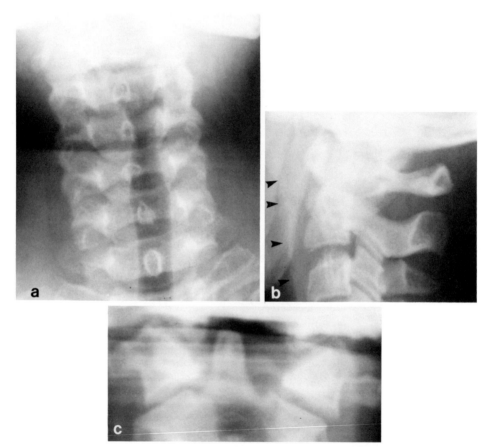

Figure 10.28. Acute traumatic rotary atlantoaxial dislocation in a young man involved in a motor-pedestrian accident. In the frontal radiograph (a) the head is tilted and the vertebrae are rotated to the left as evidenced by the relationship of the mandible to the transverse processes of T_1 and displacement of the spinous processes to the right. In the lateral projection of the cervicocranium (b), the anterior atlantodental interval is narrow and the anterior arch of the C_1 is not in true lateral projection, reflecting lateral tilt and/or rotation of the atlas on the axis. Prevertebral soft tissue swelling (arrowheads) is present. The panoramic zonogram (c) demonstrates moderately severe left lateral translation of the atlas on the axis.

As a result of rotation of the atlas, its lateral masses are displaced, one anteriorly and one posteriorly, with respect to the articular masses of C_2. These positional changes are reflected, in the frontal radiograph, by incongruity of the contiguous articulating surfaces of the atlas and axis and asymmetry of these joint spaces. The lateral atlantodental intervals become asymmetrical, as well (Fig. 10.28a). In the lateral projection, cervicocranial prevertebral soft tissue swelling is evident. Rotation of the atlas about the dens causes the anterior arch of C_1 to lose its characteristic hemispheric configuration, the anterior atlantodental interval to be indistinct, and the articular masses of C_1 to be abnormally located anterior and posterior to the dens and to the articular masses of C_2 (Fig. 10.28b).

TORTICOLLIS

While acute traumatic rotary atlantoaxial *dislocation* (discussed immediately above) is a result of a specific, identifiable incident and is associated with actual soft tissue injury, atlantoaxial rotary *displacement* (torticollis, "wry neck"), in contradistinction, usually occurs spontaneously and is not associated with a pathologic injury. The characteristic feature of atlantoaxial rotary displacement is that the relationship of the atlas to the axis is a position *normally* attained during *physiologic* rotation (157).

A review of the physiologic motions that occur in the cervicocranium during rotation and lateral bending of the head (Chapter 1, pp. 14–17) is essential to a proper evaluation of the frequently perplexing radiographic appearance of the atlantoaxial articulation in torticollis. It is unfortunate that such terms as "unilateral offset" and "bilateral offset" (158,159) have been used to describe atlantoaxial relationships that are physiologic because, through common usage, these terms have become accepted by many as indicating a pathologic condition. "Subluxation" and "dislocation" are, by definition, abnormal conditions, but the radiographic relationships of C_1–C_2 to which they have been ascribed are more often normal than abnormal. "Offset" has also, by common usage, come to be synonymous with abnormality. It has been established that unilateral offset and bilateral offset *alone* are not pathologic and should not be considered signs of subluxation or dislocation of the atlantoaxial articulation (13,66,160,161). Displacement of one or both lateral masses of the atlas in conjunction with atlantal fractures has been discussed previously. It is hoped that by describing the physiologic motions at the atlantoaxial articulation and by illustrating the roentgen appearance of these motions, the terms "offset," "rotational subluxation," and "physiologic dislocation" will be shown to be not only imprecise but frankly misleading. Fielding and Hawkins (66) have used the term "rotational displacement" to describe the physiologic changes at the atlantoaxial articulation. This term describes more accurately the events that occur during rotation and lateral bending and conveys no implication of abnormality, thus leaving the significance of the roentgen findings to interpretation in light of the clinical situation. Therefore, unless definite roentgen signs of skeletal or soft tissue injury in the cervicocranium are present, the significance of alterations in alignment of the atlas and the axis, i.e., "rotational displacement," must depend on the clinical findings.

Torticollis is a clinical condition of unknown etiology that is frequently seen in childhood and early adolescence. It usually occurs spontaneously but may also follow minor trauma to the head or neck or be associated with acute infections. It is characterized clinically by tilting of the head in one direction and simultaneous rotation of the head in the opposite direction, and is characterized radiographically by atlantoaxial rotary displacement. The pathophysiology, which is described as "locking" or "catching" (162) of the interfacetal joints at some point during physiologic rotation of the atlas on the axis, is usually self-limited and the deformity usually reverses spontaneously. Occasionally, however, the deformity may persist, in which event the altered relationship of C_1 and C_2 is referred to as atlantoaxial rotary *fixation* (66).

The roentgen evaluation of the patient with torticollis is challenging because the painful deformity makes positioning of the patient difficult and, consequently, interpretation of the roentgenograms fre-

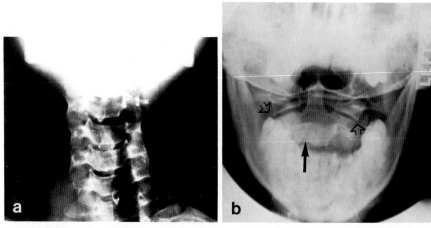

Figure 10.29. Torticollis with the head rotated and tilted to the left (*a*). In the open-mouth projection (*b*), the atlas has shifted and rotated to the left, resulting in a decrease in the width of the space between its right lateral mass and the dens (*short arrow*), an apparent increase in the transverse diameter of the right lateral mass because of its anterior rotation, and asymmetry of the lateral margins of the lateral atlantoaxial joints (*open arrows*). The left lateral mass of the axis appears truncated because of its posterior rotation. Rotation of the axis to the left is indicated by displacement of its spinous process to the right of the midline (*long arrow*).

quently perplexing. No attempt to straighten the head and neck in order to obtain a "good" (i.e., straight) anteroposterior radiograph should be attempted. To do so aggravates the patient's pain and also diminishes or eliminates the characteristic roentgen signs of torticollis. The lateral tilt and rotation of the head that occur in torticollis result in physiologic movements of the atlas and axis that have been described and illustrated in Chapter 1 (pp. 14–17). In torticollis, however, these movements are the result of the underlying etiology of the torticollis, whether it is congenital or acquired, and cannot be voluntarily reversed. The lateral tilt of the head causes the atlas to shift laterally in the same direction as the head tilt and the axis to rotate in the same direction also. The associated rotation of the head also causes the *atlas* to rotate in the same direction.

The roentgen signs of torticollis, then, are the sum of the effects of lateral tilt and rotation of the atlas and axis. Lateral tilt of C_1 causes unidirectional displacement of its articular masses with respect to the dens and those of C_2 resulting in asymmetry of the spaces between the dens and the articular masses of the axis, asymmetry of the lateral margins of the lateral atlantoaxial joints, increase in transverse diameter (width) of the anteriorly rotated articular mass of the atlas, and a displacement of the bifid spinous process of the axis from the midline in the direction opposite that of the torticollis deformity (Figs. 10.28 and 10.29). In the lateral radiograph, the rotation and lateral tilt of the atlas and axis in torticollis result in a loss of definition of the normal atlantoaxial anatomy (Fig. 10.30).

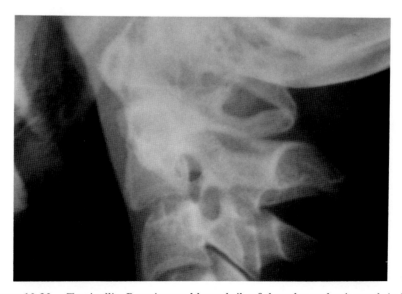

Figure 10.30. Torticollis. Rotation and lateral tilt of the atlas and axis result in loss of definition of the normal anatomy of the cervicocranium in lateral projection.

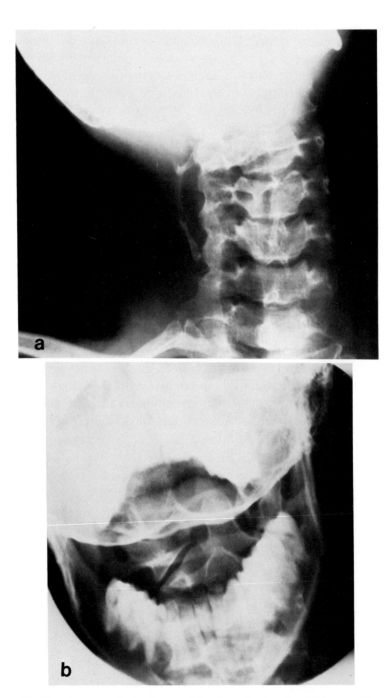

Figure 10.31. Long-standing atlantoaxial rotary fixation in a 22-year-old woman. The "wry-neck" deformity is evident in the frontal radiograph of the cervical spine (*a*) and the abnormal conformation of the atlas and axis is clearly seen in the open-mouth projection (*b*).

Atlantoaxial displacement that fails to resolve spontaneously in a few days has been termed atlantoaxial rotary *fixation* by Fielding and Hawkins (66). Persistent torticollis throughout the growing years, results in alterations in the configuration of the atlas and axis (Fig. 10.31).

SUBTLE CERVICOCRANIAL INJURIES

Having discussed occipitoatlantal disassociation and dens fractures in this chapter, it seems logical to expand that discussion to include those and other acute cervicocranial injuries that may be so subtle as to be heralded only by cervicocranial prevertebral soft tissue swelling on the initial lateral radiograph.

The evaluation of cervicocranial prevertebral soft tissue can only be subjective since no objective definitive measurements for its thickness in lateral projection have been established. A change from the normal contour or configuration of the cervicocranial prevertebral soft tissue shadow as it extends from the axis to the skull base should, with an appropriate history and physical findings, create a high index of suspicion of minimally displaced, subtle OAD (subluxation), Jefferson bursting fracture, dens fracture, or traumatic spondylolisthesis. Of all the acute injuries that can occur in the cervicocranium, these four are those most apt to be missed when minimally displaced and all are associated with cervicocranial prevertebral hemorrhage and soft tissue swelling.

Normally, the prevertebral soft tissues from the second cervical intervertebral disk space to the base of the skull generally follow the contour of the anterior cortex of the atlas and axis because this shadow represents those soft tissue structures that are densely adherent to these vertebrae, i.e., the annulus fibrosis of the related disk, the anterior atlantoaxial ligament and those that extend from the superior margin of the anterior arch of C_1 to the skull base, namely the anterior atlanto-occipital membrane and the dentate ligament and, anterior to these, the superior constrictor muscles covered by the mucosa of the posterior hypopharyngeal wall. Above the anterior arch of the atlas, the soft tissue shadow may have a slightly posterior concavity as it continues craniad to the base of the skull. Normally the posterior pharyngeal wall soft tissue-air interface is sharp (Fig. 10.32).

Hemorrhage and/or edema of the cervicocranial prevertebral soft tissues secondary to an acute cervicocranial injury causes the air-soft tissue interface to become unsharp. The contour of the soft tissue shadow changes slightly, but definitely, so that from approximately the level of the second cervical interspace upward, the soft tissue shadow becomes progressively thicker as it extends to the skull base either in an oblique (Fig. 10.18) or anteriorly convex (Fig. 10.12) curve.

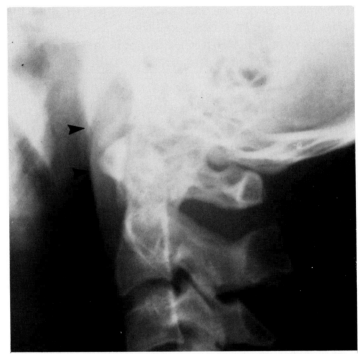

Figure 10.32.   Normal cervicocranial prevertebral soft tissue shadow (*arrowheads*).

The configuration of the soft tissue shadows cephalad to the anterior arch of C_1 may be altered by persistent adenoidal tissue which appears as a smoothly lobulated soft tissue mass extending anteriorly along the floor of the skull base toward the posterior nares. Normally, the anterior margin of the adenoidal mass is outlined by air (Fig. 10.33). Other conditions that alter or obliterate the prevertebral soft tissues include hypoventilation or breath holding in expiration (Fig. 10.34), free blood that has accumulated in the naso-oropharynx in recumbency (Fig. 10.35), swallowing during radiographic exposure, and soft tissue trauma associated with transnasal endotracheal intubation (Fig. 10.3).

Nasopharyngeal soft tissue swelling secondary to midface fractures can usually be distinguished from that secondary to cervicocranial injuries by virtue of the fact that the midface nasopharyngeal hematoma is inseparable from the midface, obliterates or obscures the posterior nares and may fill the hypopharynx, extending to and obscuring the superior surface of, and depressing, the soft palate and uvula (Fig. 10.36). This variety of nasopharyngeal hematoma extends posteriorly into the naso-oropharynx and displaces the naso-oropharyngeal

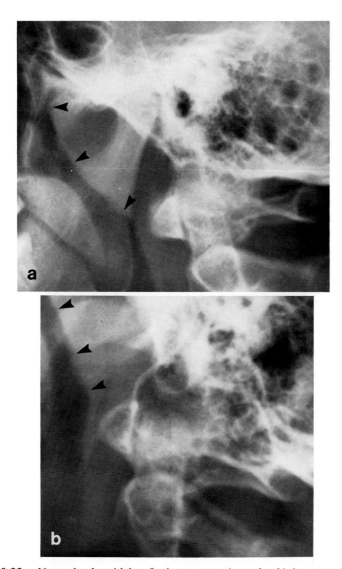

Figure 10.33. Normal adenoidal soft tissue mass (*arrowheads*) in neutral (*a*) and extended (*b*) lateral projections. The inferior surface of the mass is smoothly lobular and air is present in the nasopharynx between the anterior surface of the mass and the midfacial skeleton (*a*).

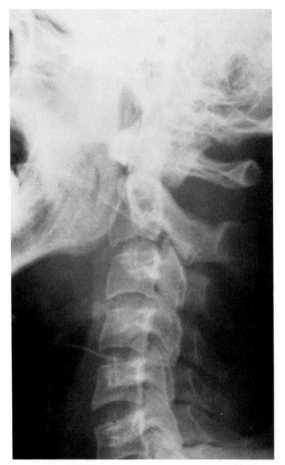

Figure 10.34. Lateral radiograph of the cervical spine with practically no air in the oro-hypopharynx. The intimate apposition of the contiguous surfaces of the base of the tongue and the posterior pharyngeal wall simulate a soft tissue mass.

mucosa anteroinferiorly, typically encroaching upon the pharygeal air space to a greater degree than does the hematoma associated with cervicocranial injury. When massive, the midface nasopharyngeal hematoma may completely occlude the oropharyngeal airway, necessitating tracheostomy.

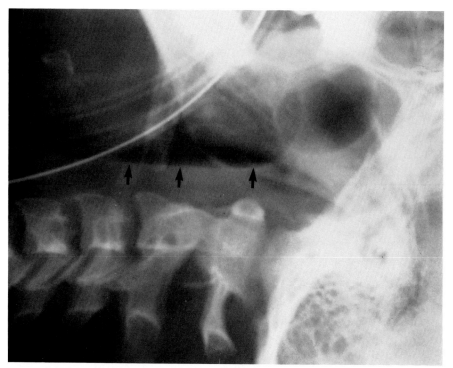

Figure 10.35. The prevertebral soft tissues are completely obscured by the free blood that has pooled in the oro-hypopharynx, of this patient examined in recumbency. The pharyngeal air-fluid level (*arrows*) indicates the accumulated blood.

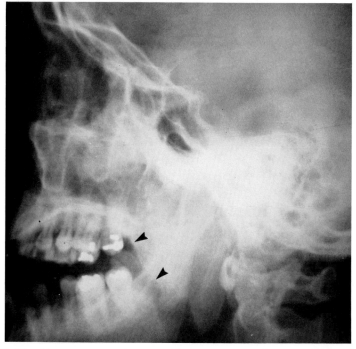

Figure 10.36. Huge naso-oropharyngeal hematoma secondary to a displaced LeFort II fracture. The soft tissue mass, which completely fills the naso-oropharynx, extends posteriorly from the midfacial skeleton and depresses the soft palate and uvula (*arrowheads*).

255

Chapter 11

Variations of Normal Anatomy that May Simulate Acute Injury

Although examples of deviations from the normal appearance of the cervical spine due to (*a*) age and normal growth and development, (*b*) positioning and radiographic technique and, (*c*) normal anatomy and normal variants have been discussed and illustrated in preceding chapters, it seems appropriate to devote one chapter to an atlas type presentation of normal variants that may simulate acute injury of the cervical spine. This is not intended to be a comprehensive review of normal variants of the muscular skeletal system. For such, the reader is referred to the recognized pertinent benchmark text (165) on the subject.

In this chapter, the figure legends constitute the text.

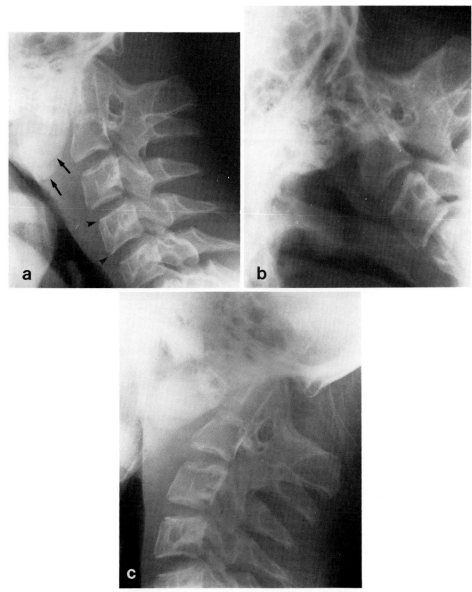

Figure 11.1. Multiple anomalies of the cervicocranium in neutral lateral (*a*), lateral flexion (*b*), and extension (*c*) projections in an adolescent patient without cervical trauma or symptoms. The anomalies include congenital posterior dislocation and fusion of the occipitoatlantal junction (occipitalization of the atlas) as well as congenital atlantoaxial fusion. The ring apophyses (*a, arrowheads*) remain ununited. The apparent cervicocranial prevertebral soft tissue mass was normal for this person, the retropharynx being negative clinically. The large globular soft tissue densities (*arrows*) represent enlarged tonsils.

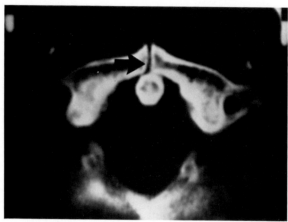

Figure 11.2.　Vertical defect of an unfused anterior arch of the atlas. The densely sclerotic, smooth margins of the defect (*arrow*) and cortical hypertrophy anteriorly are indicative of a congenital anomaly.

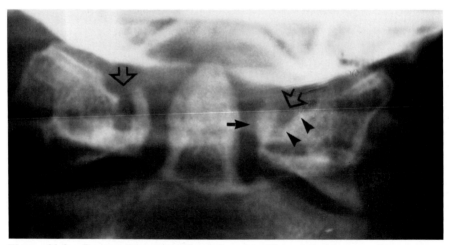

Figure 11.3.　Panoramic zonograph of the atlas. The vertical lucency (*open arrows*) between the cortex of the internal tubercle (*arrow*) and the medial cortex of the lateral mass (*arrowheads*) should not be misinterpreted for a fracture.

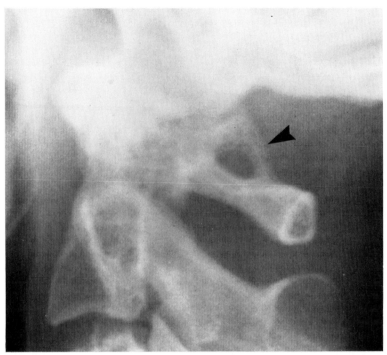

Figure 11.4.   Complete arcuate foramen (*arrowhead*) which accomodates the vertebral artery.

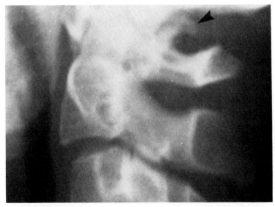

Figure 11.5.   Incomplete arcuate foramen. The corticated margins of the curved projection (*arrowhead*) forming the incomplete roof of the foramen should distinguish this
variant from a fracture.

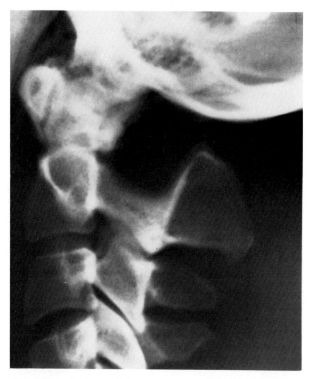

Figure 11.6. Complete absence of the posterior arch of the atlas. The spinous process of the axis is compensatorily hypertrophied.

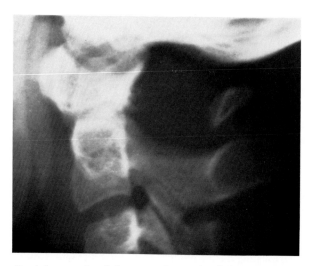

Figure 11.7. Partial agenesis of the posterior arch of the atlas. The configuration, location, and corticated margins of the posterior tubercle of the atlas should distinguish it from a fracture fragment.

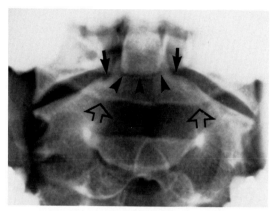

Figure 11.8.   The common variations at the junction of the base of the dens and the axis centrum (*arrows*) are illustrated in this patient. A maxillary central incisor tooth produces a negative Mach band (*arrowheads*) upon the base of the dens. The inferior cortex of the posterior arch of the atlas produces a negative Mach band (*arrowheads*) upon the base of the dens and the inferior cortex of the posterior arch of the atlas produces a positive Mach band (*open arrow*) across the axis body. Neither of the latter should be mistaken for a fracture line.

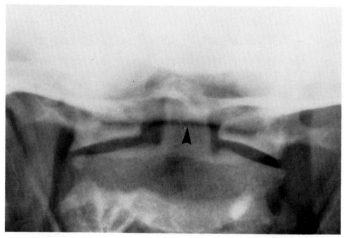

Figure 11.9.   Negative Mach band (*arrowheads*) caused by a superimposition of the occipital bone upon the dens, the lateral Atlantodentalinterval and the lateral masses of C_1.

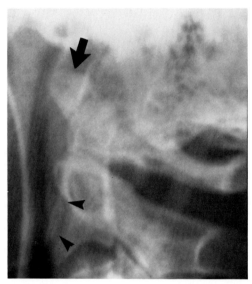

Figure 11.10.   The anterior arch of the atlas (*arrow*) appears to be cranially subluxated with respect to the dens as a result of anomalous atlantoaxial articulation. The developmental etiology of the atlantoaxial relationship in this individual may reasonably be assumed because of the hypertrophy of the anterior arch of C_1, the relative hypoplasia of the tip of the dens and the slope of its anterior surface and the absence of cervicocranial prevertebral soft tissue swelling. Superimposition of the angle of the mandible upon the body of C_2 (*arrowheads*) indicates this examination was obtained in flexion rather that extension.

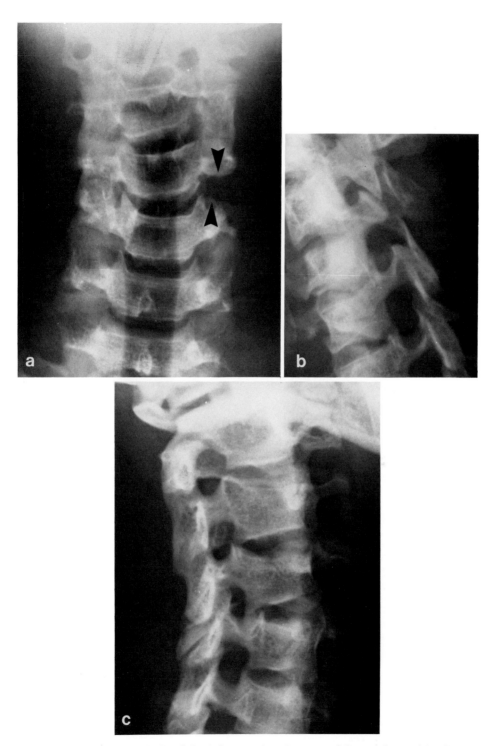

Figure 11.11. Hypoplasia of the left posterior elements of C_4 and C_5 resulting in a large defect (*arrowheads*) in the left "lateral column" (*a*). The sclerotic margins of the defect, together with the other anomalies at this level, should suggest an anomaly rather than a large fracture defect. The major anomalies of the left and the lesser anomalies of the right articular masses and laminae of C_4 and C_5 are seen to better advantage in the oblique projections (*b*) and (*c*).

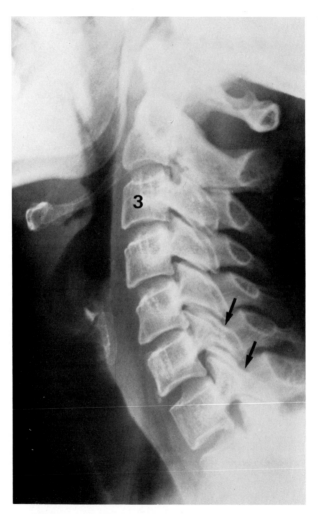

Figure 11.12.   Normal notching at the junction of the inferior margin of the superior articulating facet and C_3 and the location all bespeak anomaly rather than fracture.

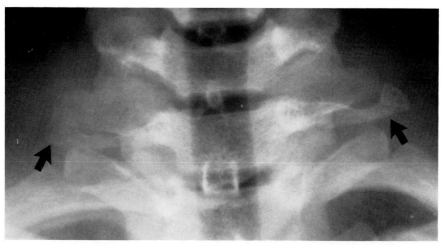

Figure 11.13 Ununited secondary ossification centers of transverse processes (*arrows*) of C₇. The bilaterality, similar appearance, and corticated margins should suggest anomaly rather than fracture.

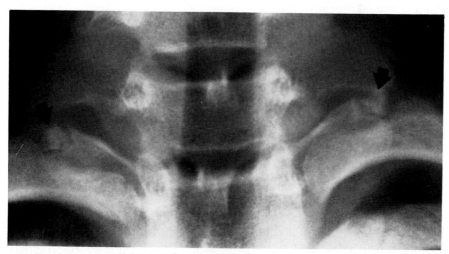

Figure 11.14 Ununited secondary ossification centers of the transverse processes of T₁ (*arrows*). The similarity, sclerotic margins of the contiguous surfaces of the secondary centers and transverse processes, and their location all bespeak anomaly rather than fracture.

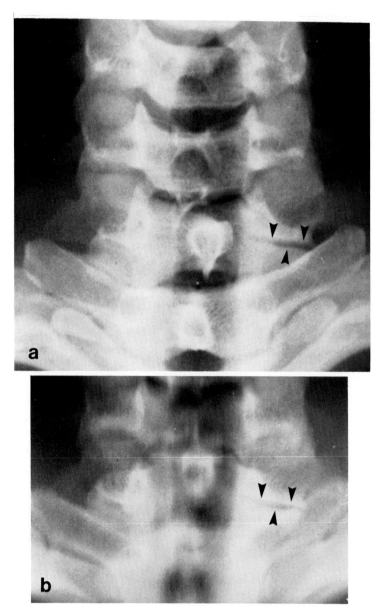

Figure 11.15.   Anomalous interfacetal joint (*arrowheads*) in the plain frontal (*a*) and rectilinear frontal tomogram (*b*) simulating an articular mass fracture. The smooth sclerotic margins of the defect are atypical for an acute fracture.

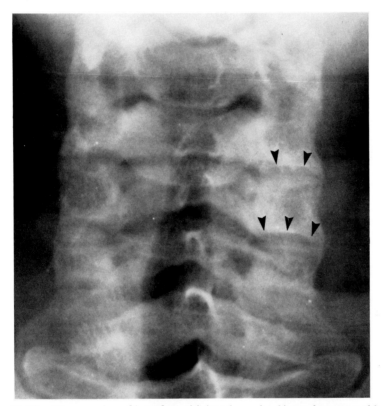

Figure 11.16. The margins of interfacetal joints (*arrowheads*) produce smoothly corticated, slightly superiorly convex or horizontal lucencies which traverse, and appear to disrupt, the "lateral column," thereby simulating fractures. The characteristics of the defects, their configuration and location, and the absence of disruption of the lateral margin of the left lateral column are all in favor of normal variation and against articular mass fracture.

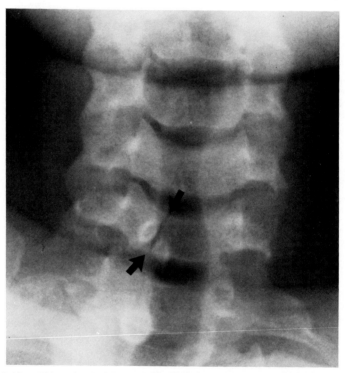

Figure 11.17.   This spina bifida occulta of C$_7$ (*arrows*) is distinguished from a posterior laminar or spinous process fracture by the smoothly corticated margin of the defect and of the bifid spinous process.

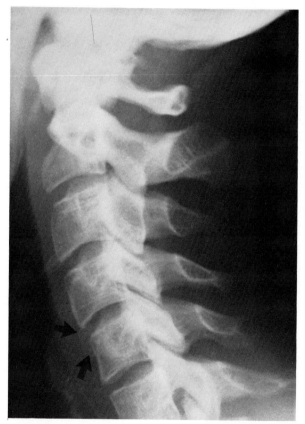

Figure 11.18.   Prominent transverse process of C₅ (*arrow*) projecting anterior to the vertebral body.

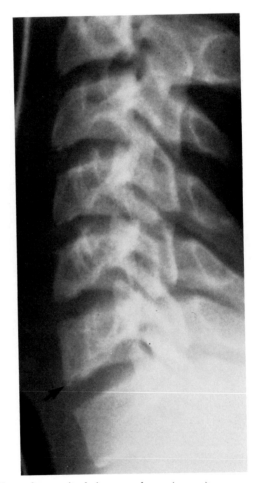

Figure 11.19.   Normal, ununited ring apophyses (*arrows*).

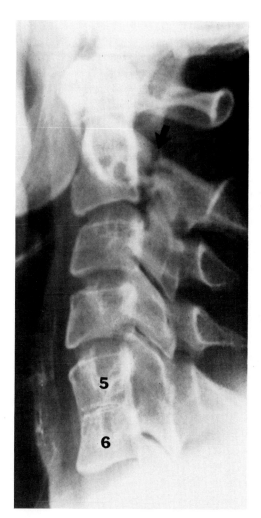

Figure 11.20. Partial congenital fusion of the bodies of C_5 and C_6 with complete fusion of their posterior elements in a patient with a Type I acute traumatic spondylolisthesis (*arrow*).

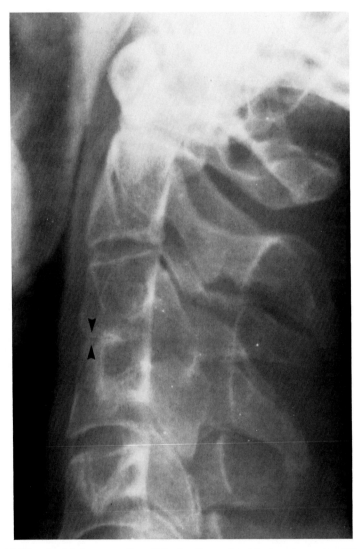

Figure 11.21.   Multiple anomalies of the bodies and posterior elements of C_3 and C_4. The thin horizontal defect of the incompletely obliterated intervertebral disk space (*arrowheads*) should not be mistaken for a fracture. The prevertebral soft tissue shadow is normal.

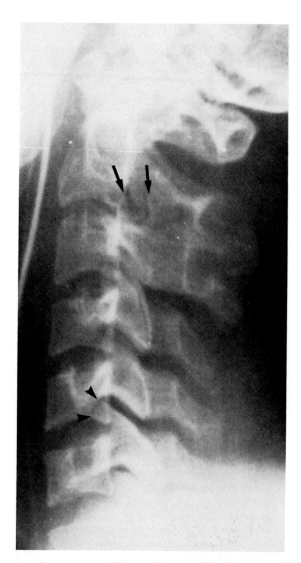

Figure 11.22. Partial congenital fusion of the posterior elements of C_2 and C_3. The anamolously oriented, rudimentary interfacetal joints of C_2–C_3 (*arrows*) should not be mistaken for a fracture line. The margins of the Mach band are smooth and extend off the centrum into the disk space.

References

1. Von Torklus, D. and Gehle, W.: The Upper Cervical Spine. Grune & Stratton, New York, 1972.
2. Schneider, R.C., Livingston, K.E., Cave, A.J.E., Hamilton, G.: "Hangman's fracture" of the cervical spine. J. Neurosurg. 22:141, 1965.
3. Bailey, R.W. (ed.): The Cervical Spine: The Cervical Spine Research Society. J.B. Lippincott Company, Philadelphia, pp 225, 226, 1983.
4. Brocker, J.E.W.: Die Occipital-Cervical-Cegend. Thieme, Stuttgart, 1955. As cited by Von Torklus & Gehle, Reference 1.
5. Locke, G.R., Gardner, J.E. & Van Epps, E.F.: Atlas-dens interval (ADI) in children. AJR 97:135, 1966.
6. Cattell, H.S. & Filtzer, D.L.: Pseudosubluxation and other normal variations of the cervical spine in children. J. Bone Joint Surg. 47-A:1295, 1965.
7. Caffey's Pediatrics X-Ray Diagnosis: An Integrated Imaging Approach. 8th Edition Edited by Fredric N. Silverman, Chicago, Yearbook Medical Publisher, 1985.
8. Swischuk, L.E.: Anterior dislocation of C_2 in children: physiologic or pathologic? Radiology 122:759, 1977.
9. Swischuk, L.E.: Emergency Radiology of the Acutely Ill or Injured Child. 2nd Edition. Williams & Wilkins, Baltimore, 1986.
10. Gray's Anatomy. 29th Ed. Philadelphia: Lea and Febiger, 1973.
11. Coutts, M.B.: Atlanto-epistropheal subluxations. Arch. Surg 29:297, 1934.
12. Fielding, J.W.: Cineroentgenography of the normal cervical spine. J. Bone Joint Surg. 39-A:1280, 1957.
13. Hohl, M.: Normal motions in the upper portion of the cervical spine. J. Bone Joint Surg. 46-A:1777, 1964.
14. Hay, P.D.: Measurement of the soft tissues of the neck. In Lusted, L.B. & Keats, T.E. (Eds.): Atlas of Roentgenographic Measurement, 3rd Ed. Chicago, Yearbook Medical Publishers, 1972.
15. Weir, D.C.: Roentgenographic signs of cervical injury. Clin. Orthop. 109:9, 1975.
16. Edeiken-Monroe, B., Wagner, L.K., & Harris, J.H., Jr.: Hyperextension dislocation of the cervical spine. AJNR 7:135, 1986.
17. Fielding, J.W.: Normal and selected abnormal motions of the cervical spine from the second cervical vertebra to the seventh cervical vertebra based on cineroentgenography. J. Bone Joint Surg. 46-A:1779, 1964.
18. White, A.A., Johnson, R.M., Panjabi, M.D., et al.: Biomedical analysis of clinical stability in the cervical spine. Clin. Orthop., 109:85, 1975.
19. Edeiken, J.: Personal communication.
20. Green, J.D., Harle, T.S., and Harris, J.H., Jr.: Anterior subluxation of the cervical spine: hyperflexion sprain. AJNR 2:243, 1981.

274

21. Holdsworth, F.: Fractures, dislocations and fracture–dislocations of the spine. J. Bone Joint Surg. 52-A:1534, 1970.
22. Kaufmann, H.H., Harris, J.H., Jr., Spencer, J.A., et al.: Danger of traction during radiography for cervical trauma. JAMA 247:2369, 1982.
23. Taylor, A.R. and Blackwood, W.: Paraplegia in cervical injuries with normal radiographic appearance. J. Bone Joint Surg. 30-B:245, 1948.
24. Miller, M.D., Gehweiler, J.A., Martinez, S., et al.: Significant new observations on cervical spine trauma. AJR 130:659, 1978.
25. Bontrager, L.B. and Anthony, B.T.: Textbook of Radiographic Positioning and Related Anatomy. Denver, Multi-Media Publishing, 1982.
26. Merrill, V.: Atlas of Roentgenographic Positions. Edition 2. St. Louis, The C.V. Mosby Company, 1959.
27. Cacayorin, E.D. and Kieffer, S.A.: Applications and limitations of computed tomography of the spine. Radiol. Clin. North Am. 20:185, 1982.
28. Ghoshhajra, K. and Rao, K.V.C.G.: CT in spinal trauma. CT 4:309, 1980.
29. Maravilla, K.R., Cooper, P.R., and Sklar, F.H.: The influence of thin-section tomography on the treatment of cervical spine injuries. Radiology 127:131, 1978.
30. Trunkey, D.D. & Margulis, A.R.: Foreword in Federle, M., and Brandt-Zawadski, M. (eds.): Computed Tomography in the Evaluation of Trauma. Baltimore, Williams & Wilkins, 1982.
31. Angtuaco, E.J.C. and Binet, E.F.: Radiology of thoracic and lumbar fractures. Clin. Orthop., 189:43, 1984.
32. Keene, J.S., Goletz, T.H., Lilleas, F., et al.: Diagnosis of vertebral fractures: a comparison of conventional radiography, conventional tomography and computed axial tomography. J. Bone Joint Surg. 64-A:586–595, 1982.
33. Wojcik, W.G. and Harris, J.H. Jr., "Three dimensional CT scanning in the evaluation of acute spinal trauma." Radiology 157(p):236, 1985.
34. Brandt-Zawadski, M. and Minagi, H.: CT in the Evaluation of Spine Trauma: Computed Tomography in the Evaluation of Trauma. Baltimore, Williams & Wilkins, 1982.
35. Kaufman, B.: Metrizamide enhanced computed tomography and newer techniques of myelography. In Baliley, R.W., Sherk, H.H., Dunn, E.J., et al. (eds.): The Cervical Spine. Philadelphia, J.B. Lippincott Company, 1983, pp 103–111.
36. Yeakley, J., Edeiken-Monroe, B., and Harris, J.H., Jr.: Computed tomography of spinal trauma and degenerative disease. AAOS Instr. Course Lect., 1985.
37. Federle, M. and Brandt-Zawadski, M. (eds.): Computed Tomography in the Evaluation of Trauma. Baltimore, Williams & Wilkins, 1982.
38. Post, J.D. (ed): Radiographic Evaluation of the Spine: Current Advances with Emphasis on Computed Tomography. Masson Publishing, U.S.A., Inc., 1980.
39. Leo, J. S., Bergeron, R.T., Kricheff, I.I., et al.: Metrizamide myelography for cervical spinal cord injuries. Radiology 129:707, 1978.
40. McGahan, J.P., Benson, D., et al.: Intraoperative sonographic monitoring of reduction spinal fractures. Abstract presented at Radiological Society of North America Scientific Assembly, Washington, D.C., 1984.
41. Apley, A.G.: Fracture of the spine. Ann. R. Coll. Surg. Engl., 46:210, 1970.
42. Babcock, J.L.: Cervical spine injuries: diagnosis and classification. Arch. Surg., 111:646, 1976.
43. Beatson, T.R.: Fractures and dislocations of the cervical spine. J. Bone Joint Surg. [Br.], 45:21, 1963.
44. Bedbrook, G.M.: Spinal injuries with tetraplegia and paraplegia. J. Bone Joint Surg. [Br.], 61:267, 1979.
45. Braakman, R., and Penning, L.: Injuries of the Cervical Spine. Amsterdam, Excerpta Medica, 1971.
46. Gehweiler, J.A., Jr., Clar, W.M., Schaaf, R.E., et al.: Cervical spine trauma: the common combined conditions. Radiology, 130:77, 1979.

47. Holdsworth, F.: Fractures, dislocations and fracture-dislocations of the spine. J. Bone Joint Surg. [Br.], 45:6, 1963.
48. King, D.M.: Fractures and dislocations of the cervical part of the spine. Aust. N.Z. J. Surg., 37:57, 1967.
49. Maroon, J.C., Steele, P.B., and Berlin, R.: Football head and neck injuries–an update. Clin. Neurosurg., pp. 414–429.
50. Roaf, R.: A study of the mechanics of spinal injuries. J. Bone Joint Surg. [Br.], 42:810, 1960.
51. Selecki, B.R., and Williams, H.B.L.: Injuries to the Cervical Spine and Cord in Man. Australian Medical Association. Mervyn Archdall Medical Monograph Number 7, New South Wales, Australasian Medical Publishing Co., 1970.
52. Whitley, J.E., and Forsyth, H.F.: The classification of cervical spine injuries. A.J.R., 83:633, 1960.
53. Bauze, R.J., and Ardran, G.M.: Experimental production of forward dislocation in the human cervical spine. J. Bone Joint Surg. [Br.], 60:239, 1978.
54. Gosch, H.H., Gooding, E., and Schneider, R.C.: An experimental study of cervical spine and cord injuries. J. Trauma, 12:570, 1972.
55. White, A.A., III, and Panjabi, M.M.: Clinical Biomechanics of the Spine. Philadelphia, J.B. Lippincott, 1978.
56. Marar, B.C.: The pattern of neurological damage as an aid to the diagnosis of the mechanism of cervical spine injuries. J. Bone Joint Surg. [Am.], 56:1648, 1974.
57. Taylor, A.R.: The mechanism of injury to the spinal cord in the neck without damage to the vertebral column. J. Bone Joint Surg. [Br.], 39:543, 1951.
58. Louis, R.: Surgery of the Spine: Surgical Anatomy and Operative Approaches. Berlin, Springer–Verlag, 1983.
59. Panjabi, M.M., White, A.A., and Johnson, R.M.: Cervical spine mechanics as a function of transection of components. J. Biomech., 8:327, 1975.
60. Denis, F.: The three column spine and its significance in the classification of acute thoracolumbar spinal injuries. Spine, 8:817, 1983.
61. Allen, B.L., Ferguson, R.L., Lehman, T.R., et al.: A mechanistic classification of closed, indirect fractures and dislocations of the lower cervical spine. Spine, 7:1, 1982.
62. Gehweiler, J.A., Osborne, R.L., and Becker, R.F.: The Radiology of Vertebral Trauma. Volume 16. Saunders Monographs in Clinical Radiology. Philadelphia, W. B. Saunders Company, 1980.
63. Cheshire, D.J.: The stability of the cervical spine following the conservative treatment of fractures and fracture-dislocations. Paraplegia, 7:193, 1969.
64. Cramer, F., and McGowan, F.J.: The role of the nucleus pulposus in the pathogenesis of so called "recoil" injuries of the spinal cord. Surg. Gynecol. Obstet., 79:516, 1944.
65. Evans, D.K.: Anterior cervical subluxation. J. Bone Joint Surg. [Br.], 58:318, 1976.
66. Fielding, J.W., and Hawkins, R.J.: Roentgen diagnosis of the injured neck. AAOS Instr. Course Lect., 25:149, 1976.
67. Harris, J.H., Jr.: The Radiology of Acute Cervical Spine Trauma. First Edition. Baltimore, Williams & Wilkins, 1978.
68. Hohl, M.: Soft–tissue injuries of the neck in automobile accident. J. Bone Joint Surg. [Am.], 56:1675, 1974.
69. Jackson, R.: Up–dating the neck. Trauma, 1:9, 1970.
70. Kerwalramani, L.S., and Taylor, R.G.: Injuries to the cervical spine from diving accidents. Trauma, 15:130, 1975.
71. Rogers, W.A.: Fractures and dislocations of the cervical spine. J. Bone Joint Surg. [Am.], 39:341, 1957.
72. Scher, A.T.: Anterior cervical subluxation: an unstable position. A.J.R., 133:275, 1979.

73. Stringa, G.: Traumatic lesions of the cervical spine—statistics, mechanism, classification. In Proceedings of the IXth Congress of the International Society of Orthopedic Surgeons and Traumatology. Brussels, Imprimerie des Sciences, 1963, pp. 69–97.

74. Taylor, R.G., and Gleave, J.R.W.: Injuries to the cervical spine. Proc. R. Soc. Med., 55:1053, 1962.

75. Webb, J.K., Broughton, R.B.J., McSweeney, T., et al.: Hidden flexion injury of the cervical spine. J. Bone Joint Surg. [Br.], 58:322, 1976.

76. Cancelmo, J.J., Jr.: Clay shoveler's fracture: a helpful diagnostic sign. A.J.R., 115:540, 1972.

77. O'Brien, P.J., Schweigel, J.F., and Thompson, W.J.: Dislocations of the lower cervical spine. J. Trauma, 22:710, 1982.

78. Pick, R.Y., and Segal, D.: C7;-T1 bilateral facet dislocation. Clin. Orthop., 150:131, 1980.

79. Scher, A.T.: Vertex impact and cervical dislocation in rugby players. S. Afr. Med. J., 59:227, 1981.

80. Sonntag, V.K.H.: Management of bilateral locked facets of the cervical spine. Neurosurgery, 8:150, 1981.

81. American Spinal Cord Injury Association: Appendix: American Spinal Injury Association Nomenclature. In Post, M.J.D.: Radiographic Evaluation of the Spine. New York, Masson Publishing U.S.A., 1980, pp. 692–693.

82. Mazur, J.M., and Stauffer, E.S.P Unrecognized spinal instability associated with seemingly "simple" cervical compression fractures. Spine, 8:687, 1983.

83. Herrick, R.T.: Clay–shoveler's fracture in power–lifting: a case report. Am. J. Sports Med., 9:29, 1981.

84. Schneider, R.C.: Cervical spine and spinal cord injuries. Mich. Med., November 1964, pp. 773–786.

85. Schneider, R.C., and Kahn, E.A.: Chronic neurological sequelae of acute trauma to the spine and spinal cord. Part 1. The significance of the acute–flexion or "teardrop" fracture–dislocation of the cervical spine. J. Bone Joint Surg. [Am.], 38:985, 1956.

86. Schneider, R.C.: The syndrome of acute anterior spinal cord injury. J. Neurosurg., 12:95, 1955.

87. Bohlman, H.H.: Acute fractures and dislocations of the cervical spine—an analysis of three hundred hospitalized patients and review of the literature. J. Bone Joint Surg. [Am.], 61:1119, 1979.

88. Braakman, R., and Vinken, P.J.: Unilateral facet interlocking in the lower cervical spine. J. Bone Joint Surg. [Br.], 49:249, 1967.

89. Door, L.D., and Harvey, J.P., Jr.: The traumatic lesions in fatal acute spinal column injuries. Clin. Orthop., 157:178, 1981.

90. Rorabeck, C.H., Bourne, R.B., Hawkins, R.J., et al.: Unilateral facet dislocation of the cervical spine: diagnosis and results of treatment. (Abstract.) J. Bone Joint Surg. [Br.], 64:641, 1982.

91. Scher, A.T.: Unilateral locked facet in cervical spine injuries. A.J.R., 129:45, 1976.

92. Miller, M.D., Gehweiler, J.A., Martinez, S., et al.: Significant new observations on cervical spine trauma. A.J.R., 130:659, 1978.

93. Scher, A.T.: Articular pillar fractures of the cervical spine: diagnosis on the anteroposterior radiograph. S. Afr. Med. J., 60:968, 1981.

94. Smith, R.G., Beckley, D.E., and Abel, M.S.: Articular mass fracture: A neglected cause of post–traumatic pain? Clin. Radiol., 27:335, 1976.

95. Vines, F.S.: The significance of "occult" fractures of the cervical spine. A.J.R., 107:493, 1969.

96. Woodring, J.H., and Goldstein, S.J.: Fractures of the articular processes of the cervical spine. A.J.R., 139:341, 1982.

97. Jefferson, G.: Fracture of the atlas vertebra. Report of four cases, and a review of those previously recorded. Br. J. Surg., 7:407, 1920.
98. Kazarian, L.: Injuries to the human spinal column. Exerc. Sport Sci. Rev., 9:297, 1981.
99. Rothman, R.H., and Simeone, F.A.: The Spine. Philadelphia, W. B. Saunders Company, 1975.
100. Feuer, H.: Management of acute spine and spinal cord injuries. Old and new concepts. Arch. Surg., 111:638, 1976.
101. Garber, W.N., Fischer, R.G., and Holfman, H.W.: Vertebrectomy and fusion for "tear–drop fracture" of the cervical spine: case report. J. Trauma, 9:887, 1969.
102. Petrie, J.G.: Flexion injuries of the cervical spine. J. Bone Joint Surg. [Am.], 46:1800, 1964.
103. Scher, A.T.: "Tear-drop" fractures of the cervical spine—radiological features. S. Afr. Med. J., 61:355, 1981.
104. orovich, B., Peyser, E., and Gruskiewicz, J.: Acute central and intermediate cervical cord injury (Case V). Neurochirurgia, 21:77, 1978.
105. Cintron, E., Gilula, L.A., Murphy, W.A., et al.: The widened disk space: a sign of cervical hyperextension injury. Radiology, 141:639, 1981.
106. Fruin, A.H., and Pirotte, T.P.: Traumatic atlantoocipital dislocation: case report. J. Neurosurg., 46:663, 1977.
107. Harris, W.H., Hamblen, D.L., and Ojemann, R.G.: Traumatic disruption of cervical intervertebral disk from hyperextension injury. Clin. Orthop., 60:163, 1968.
108. MacNab, I.: Acceleration injuries of the cervical spine. J. Bone Joint Surg. [Am.], 46:1797, 1964.
109. Marar, B.C.: Hyperextension injuries of the cervical spine—the pathogenesis of damage to the spinal cord. J. Bone Joint Surg. [Am.], 56:1655, 1974.
110. Gehweiler, J.A., Duff, D.E., Martinez, S., et al.: Fractures of the atlas vertebra. Skeletal Radiol., 1:97, 1976.
111. Von Torklus, D., and Gehle, W.: The Upper Cervical Spine. New York, Grune & Stratton, 1972, pp. 45–48.
112. Shapiro, R., Youngberg, A.S., and Rothman, S.L.: The differential diagnosis of traumatic lesions of the occipito–atlanto–axial segment. Radiol. Clin. North Am., 11:505, 1973.
113. Sherk, H.H., and Nicholson, J.T.: Fractures of the atlas. J. Bone Joint Surg. [Am.], 52:1017, 1968.
114. Shrago, G.G.: Cervical spine injuries: association with head trauma. A review of 50 patients. A.J.R., 118:670, 1973.
115. Sinbert, J.E., and Berman, M.S.: Fracture of the posterior arch of the atlas. J.A.M. A., 114:1996, 1940.
116. Scher, A.T.: Cervical laminar fractures radiological identification. S. Afr. Med. J., 59:76, 1981.
117. Scher, A.T.: Diversity of radiologic features in hyperextension injury of the cervical spine. S. Afr. Med. J., 58:27, 1980.
118. Cornish, B.L.: Traumatic spondylolisthesis of the axis. J. Bone Joint Surg. [Br.], 50:31, 1968.
119. Effendi, B., Roy, D., Cornish, B., et al.: Fractures of the ring of the axis: a classification based on the analysis of 131 cases. J. Bone Joint Surg. [Br.], 63:319, 1981.
120. Elliott, J.M., Jr., Rogers, L.F., Wessinger, J.P., et al.: Than hangman's fracture. Radiology, 104:303, 1972.
121. Forsyth, H.F.: Extension injuries of the cervical spine. J. Bone Joint Surg. [Am.], 46:1792, 1964.
122. Roaf, R.: Spinal deformity and paraplegia. Paraplegia, 2:112, 1964.
123. Schaaf, R.E., Gehweiler, J.A., Jr., Miller, M.D., et al.: Lateral hyperflexion injuries of the spine. Skeletal Radiol., 3:73, 1978.

124. Bucholz, R.W., and Burkhead, W.Z.: The pathological anatomy of fatal atlanto-occipital dislocations. J. Bone Joint Surg. [Am.], 61:248, 1979.
125. Dublin, A.B., Marks, W.M., Weinstock, D., et al.: Traumatic dislocation of the atlanto–occipital articulation (AOA) with short–term survival with a radiographic method of measuring the AOA. J. Neurosurg., 52:541, 1980.
126. Eismont, F.J., and Bohlman, H.H.: Posterior atlanto–occipital dislocation with fractures of the atlas and odontoid process: report of a case survival. J. Bone Joint Surg. [Am.], 60:397, 1978.
127. Gabrielsen, T.O., and Maxwell, J.A.: Traumatic atlantooccipital dislocation with case report of a patient who survived. A.J.R., 97:624, 1966.
128. oodring, J.H., Selke, A.C., Jr., and Duff, D.E.: Traumatic atlantooccipital dislocation with survival. A.J.R., 137:21, 1981.
129. Powers, B., Miller, M.D., Dramer, R.S., et al.: Traumatic anterior atlanto–occipital dislocation. Neurosurgery, 4:12, 1979.
130. Southwick, W.O.: Management of fractures of the dens (odontoid process). J. Bone Joint Surg. [Am.], 62:482, 1980.
131. Anderson, L.D., and D'Alonzo, R. T.: Fractures of the odontoid process of the axis. J. Bone Joint Surg. [Am.], 56:1663, 1974.
132. Alexander, E., Jr., Forsyth, H.F., Davis, C.H., et al.: Dislocation of the atlas on the axis. The value of early fusion of C1, C2, and C3. J. Neurosurg., 15:353, 1958.
133. Harris, J.H., Jr., Burke, J.T., Ray, R.D., et al.: Low (Type III) odontoid fracture: a new radiologic sign. Radiology, 153:353, 1984.
134. Braakman, R, Penning, L.: The hyperflexion sprain of the cervical spine. Radiol Clin Biol 37:309, 1968.
135. Dosch, J.C.: Trauma: Conventional Radiological Study in Spine Injury. New York, Springer-Verlag, 1985.
136. Bedbrook, G.M.: Stability of spinal fractures and fracture dislocations. Paraplegia 9:23, 1971.
137. Jofe, M.H, White, A.A., Panjabi, M.M.: Physiology and Biomechanics: kinematics. Chapter 2, pp.23–35 In: The Cervical Spine. Ed. The Cervical Spine Research Society. J.B. Lippincott, Philadelphia, 1983.
138. Rogers, L.F.: Radiology of Skeletal Trauma. Churchill Livingstone, New York, NY, 1982.
139. Penning, L: Roentgenographic Evaluation: Obtaining and interpreting Plain Films in Cervical Spine Injury. In: The Cervical Spine. Ed: The Cervical Spine Research Society. J.B. Lippincott, Philadelphia, 1983.
140. Schneider, R.C.: A syndrome in acute cervical spine injuries for which early operation is indicated. J Neurosurg 8:360, 1951.
141. Fielding, J.W., Cochran, G.V.B., Lawsing, J.F. III and Hohl, M: Tears of the transverse ligament of the atlas. J Bone Surg 56-A:1683, 1974.
142. Lee, C., Kim, K.S., Rogers, L.F.,: Sagittal fracture of the cervical vertebral body. AJR 139:55–60, 1982.
143. Garber, J.N.: Abnormalities of the atlas and axis vertebrae—congenital and traumatic. J Bone Joint Surg. 46-A:1792, 1964.
144. Francis, W.R., Fielding, R.J., Pepin, J. and Hensinger, R.: Traumatic spondylolisthesis of the axis. J Bone Joint Surg 63-B:313–318, 1981.
145. Harris, W., Hamblen, D., Ojemann, R.: Traumatic disruption of cervical intervertebral disc from hyperextension injury. Clin Orthop 60:163–167, 1968.
146. Levine, A.M. and Edwards, C.C.: The management of traumatic spondylolosthesis of the axis. J Bone Joint Surg 67-A:217–226, 1985.
147. Courville, C.B.: Pathology of the Central Nervous System. Pacific Press Publishing Assn., Mountain View, CA., 1937.
148. Watson-Jones R.: Journal of Bone and Joint Surgery 20:567, 1938.
149. Pendergrass E.P., Shaeffer, J.P. and Hodes, P.J.: The head and neck in roentgen diagnosis. Charles C. Thomas. Springfield, IL., 1956.

150. Wilson, P.D. and Cochran WA: Fractures and Dislocations: Ed 2. Philadelphia. J.B. Lippincott Company, 1929.

151. Mixter, W.J.: Fracture and Dislocation of the Spine. Nelson's Looseleaf Surgery. New York and London, Thos. Nelson and Son, Vol. III, Chapter 12, pp. 871, 1941.

152. Schatzker, J., Rorabeck, C.H. and Waddell, J.P.: Fractures of the dens (odontoid process); an analysis of 37 cases. J Bone Joint Surg 53-B:392, 1971.

153. Fielding, J.W. and Griffin, P.P.: Os odontoideum: an acquired lesion. J Bone Joint Surg 56-A:187, 1974.

154. El-Khoury, G.Y., Clark, C.R. and Graveth, A.W.: Acute traumatic rotary atlantoaxial dislocation in three children. J Bone Joint Surg 66-A:774-777, 1984.

155. Corner, E.M.: Rotary dislocations of the atlas. Ann Surg 45:9–26, 1907.

156. Greeley, P.W.: Bilateral (ninety degrees) rotary dislocation of the atlas upon the axis. J Bone Joint Surg 12:958–962, 1930.

157. Wortzman, G. and Dewar, F.P.: Rotary affixation of the atlanto-axial joint: rotational atlanto-axial subluxation. Rad 90:479-487, 1986.

158. Jacobson, G. and Alder, D.C: An evaluation of lateral atlanto-axial displacement in injuries of the cervical spine. Radiology 61:355, 1961.

159. Jacobson, G. and Alder, D.C.: Examination of the atlanto-axial joint following injury with particular emphasis on rotational subluxation. AJR 76:1081, 1956.

160. Paul, L.W., and Moir, W.W.: Non-pathologic variations in relationship of the upper cervical vertebrae. Radiology 62:519, 1949.

161. Hohl, M. and Baker, H.R.: The atlanto-axial joint. J Bone Joint Surg 46-A:1739, 1964.

162. Schmorl, G. and Junghanns, H.: The Human Spine in Health and Disease, 2nd Am. Ed. Grune and Stratton, New York, NY, 1971.

163. Nichols-Hostetter, S., Ray, R., Burke, J., Harris, J.H., Jr.: Acute traumatic injuries of the axis. Presented at the the 83rd annual meeting of the American Roentgen Ray Society, Atlanta, GA., April 18–22, 1983.

164. Burke, J.T.: Personal communication. "Review of 50 patients with atlas fractures.

165. Hostetter et al: Personal communication.

166. Keats, T.E.: An Atlas of Normal Variants that May Simulate Disease. Year Book Medical Publishers. Chicago, IL, 1984.

167. Garfin, S.R. and Rothmann, R.H.: Traumatic spondylolisthesis of axis, in: The Cervical Spine, p. 223–232. Philadelphia, J.B. Lippincott, 1983.

168. Sherk, H.H. and Howard, T.: Clinical and pathologic correlations in traumatic spondylolisthesis of the axis. Clin. Orthop, 174:122–126, 1983.

169. Francis, W.R. and Fielding, J.W.: Traumatic spondylolisthesis of the axis. Orthop. Clin North Am., 9:1011–1027, 1978.

Index

Page numbers in *italics* denote figures;
those followed by "t" denote tables.